Habits: Remaking

Habits: Remaking Addiction

Suzanne Fraser
National Drug Research Institute, Curtin University, Australia

David Moore
National Drug Research Institute, Curtin University, Australia

and

Helen Keane
School of Sociology, Australian National University, Australia

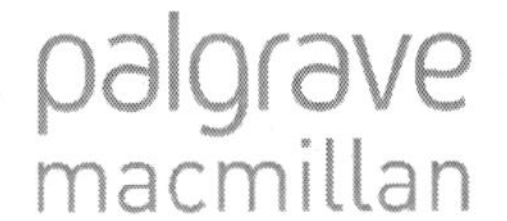

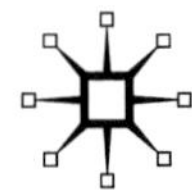

Softcover reprint of the hardcover 1st edition 2014 978-0-230-30810-7

First published 2014 by
PALGRAVE MACMILLAN

Palgrave Macmillan in the UK is an imprint of Macmillan Publishers Limited, registered in England, company number 785998, of Houndmills, Basingstoke, Hampshire RG21 6XS.

Palgrave Macmillan in the US is a division of St Martin's Press LLC, 175 Fifth Avenue, New York, NY 10010.

Palgrave Macmillan is the global academic imprint of the above companies and has companies and representatives throughout the world.

Palgrave® and Macmillan® are registered trademarks in the United States, the United Kingdom, Europe and other countries.

ISBN 978-1-349-33888-7   ISBN 978-1-137-31677-6 (eBook)

DOI 10.1057/9781137316776

A catalogue record for this book is available from the British Library.

A catalog record for this book is available from the Library of Congress.

Transferred to Digital Printing in 2014

Contents

Figures and Tables

Figure

Tables

Acknowledgements

This book is partly based on three research projects funded by Australia's national competitive grant bodies, the Australian Research Council and the National Health and Medical Research Council (details in the Appendix). We would like to acknowledge this support and note the value of such schemes in helping make possible large-scale sociological research of the kind reflected in this book. The authors were based at two institutions: the National Drug Research Institute (NDRI), Faculty of Health Sciences, Curtin University and the College of Arts and Social Sciences, Australian National University (ANU). The NDRI is supported by funding from the Australian Government under the Substance Misuse Prevention and Service Improvement Grants Fund. We are grateful for the support we received from our colleagues during the process of writing this book. We are also grateful to Sweden's alcohol and other drug research centre, SoRAD, based at Stockholm University, for acting as hosts during the month we enjoyed as visiting scholars in 2013.

Of course, each of us also drew support and inspiration from different sources, and our individual acknowledgements appear below.

Suzanne Fraser This book was made possible by the intelligence, skill and perseverance of my co-authors, David Moore and Helen Keane. It has been an absolute pleasure to work with them on this ambitious project, and I look forward to more collaboration in the future. Over the last two years, I have spent time at the National Centre in HIV Social Research (now CSRH) UNSW, where I am a visiting senior research fellow, as well as at NDRI, and I thank the staff at both centres for their collegiality and friendship. To my remarkable family I extend my warmest thanks for their indispensable support.

David Moore I'm extremely grateful for the opportunity to collaborate with co-authors Suzanne Fraser and Helen Keane. I can't think of two people I'd rather work with – their acute insights, exceptional generosity and (frankly incomprehensible) modesty make them ideal research colleagues. I thank my colleagues – at NDRI and beyond – for their support and interest. And special thanks to Suzanne, Joe and Charlie for everything else.

Helen Keane Deep-felt thanks to Suzanne Fraser and David Moore for inviting me onto this project. Working with them has been intellectually rewarding *and* a genuine uncomplicated pleasure. I'd especially like to acknowledge Suzanne's efficient and thoughtful project management. Completion of the manuscript was enabled by a visiting fellowship at the NDRI, Curtin University, and a semester's research leave provided by the College of Arts and Social Sciences, ANU. I am grateful for the collegiality and friendship of my colleagues at the School of Sociology, ANU. My thanks as always to Daniel, Leon and Julius for their love and encouragement.

General

Parts of the chapters to follow have already appeared in print. We are pleased to acknowledge the publishers' permission to include them. Sections of Chapter 1 appeared in Keane, H. (2012) Diagnosing drug problems and the DSM. *Contemporary Drug Problems*, 39(3): 353–371, and are reproduced with permission from Federal Legal Publications. Tables 1 and 2 in Chapter 1 are reproduced from the *Diagnostic and Statistical Manual of Mental Disorders DSM-IV-TR* and the *Diagnostic and Statistical Manual of Mental Disorders DSM-5*, with permission from the American Psychiatric Association. Sections of Chapter 3 appeared in Fraser, S. and Moore, D. (2011). Governing through problems: The formulation of policy on amphetamine-type stimulants (ATS) in Australia. *International Journal of Drug Policy*, 22(6): 498–506, and are reproduced with permission from Elsevier. Figure 1 in Chapter 4 appeared in Ducci, F. & Goldman, D. (2008). Genetic approaches to addiction: Genes and alcohol. *Addiction*, 103: 1414–1428, and is reproduced with permission from Wiley. Sections of Chapter 6 appeared in Fraser, S. (2013). Junk: Overeating and obesity and the neuroscience of addiction. *Addiction Research & Theory*, 19(2): 230–244.

Abbreviations

ANCD	Australian National Council on Drugs
AOD	alcohol and other drug
APA	American Psychiatric Association
ATS	amphetamine-type stimulants
BMI	body mass index
BPS	British Psychological Society
CBT	cognitive behavioural therapy
CIDI	composite international diagnostic interview
DSM	Diagnostic and Statistical Manual of Mental Disorders
ED	emergency department
MCDS	Ministerial Council on Drug Strategy (Australia)
MMT	methadone maintenance treatment
NDARC	National Drug and Alcohol Research Centre (Australia)
NIAAA	National Institute on Alcohol Abuse and Alcoholism (USA)
NIDA	National Institute on Drug Abuse (USA)
NIMH	National Institute of Mental Health (USA)
NRT	nicotine replacement therapy
OCD	obsessive-compulsive disorder
OFC	orbitofrontal cortex
ONDCP	Office of National Drug Control Policy (USA)
PET	positron emission tomography
SAmDQ	Severity of Amphetamine Dependence Questionnaire
SDS	Severity of Dependence Scale
STS	science and technology studies
SUD	substance use disorder
UNDCP	United Nations Drug Control Programme
WHO	World Health Organization

Introduction

What is 'addiction'? What does it say about us, our social arrangements and our political preoccupations? Where is it going as an idea, and what is at stake in its ongoing production? These are the questions this book seeks to answer. Fuelled by recent debates about the newly published and controversial fifth edition of the *Diagnostic and Statistical Manual of Mental Disorders* (*DSM-5* 2013), by the rise of neuroscience and by the ever-increasing concern over newly defined areas of 'compulsive behaviour' or 'process addictions' (gambling, Internet and video gaming, eating and so on), the currency of the term can only be said to be growing. As Eve Sedgwick (1993) once said, an epidemic of 'addiction attribution' is underway. Our focus in this book will be on understandings of drug addiction. Perhaps the most feared of all addiction attributions, drug addiction occupies a key place in the logic of addiction. Potent substances are understood to cause harmful psychological or, more recently, neurobiological states and, in turn, problematic, often criminal – certainly destructive – behaviour. It follows that we must act to reduce the availability of drugs, our desire for them and their negative effects wherever we can. We must turn to science to help us understand drugs and addiction objectively and to lead the way in responding to the profound social problem of addiction.

Of course, the action of drugs and the meaning of addiction are far more complex than this commonplace formulation suggests. Drugs have all sorts of effects, and addiction turns out to be far less stable and predictable than we tend to believe. This instability is particularly evident when we trace these terms across different substances, and in this book we intend to do just that. Taking our lead from the recent widespread upsurge in concern about methamphetamine ('crystal meth' or 'ice') and changing conventions around alcohol consumption, as healthy drinking recommendations are becoming ever-more conservative, we track the changing meanings of addiction, identifying shifts and continuities entailed in these developments. How is addiction remade in debates about methamphetamine and alcohol? How might the primary source of accepted wisdom on drugs – scientific knowledge – be contributing to these definitions? Are there points at which the sciences inadvertently undo their own certainties about drugs and addiction? In particular, how should we understand the continuing growth in the number of substances defined as 'drugs'? Most notable among these new drugs must be food. Food, it turns out (for now), changes our brain chemistry and therefore our perceptions and behaviour. It can compromise our health and well-being even as it fulfils our most basic needs. In a strikingly familiar narrative, vulnerable people (or brains) collide with powerful, compelling substances (not crack here, nor heroin or ice, but potato chips, chocolate biscuits and white bread. Frozen pizza. Ice cream. The stuff of every once-respectable home). This rather remarkable development in the composition of 'drugs' demands examination, especially in tandem with the major developments in ideas of addiction also underway in relation to methamphetamine and alcohol. For this reason, we have chosen to include the emerging idea of food addiction in this book.

As will become clearer throughout the book, 'addiction' tells us much more about ourselves than even the most ambitious confessional, evangelical, recovery discourses articulate. Addiction and modern societies have, we insist, *made each other, and they continue to rely upon each other for meaning* (Fraser & Moore 2011). As the boundaries, contents and shapes of addictions are remade anew in emerging battles over stimulant psychosis, binge drinking and obesity, so too are the subjects and practices of modern societies. As addiction grows and changes, so do we, whether addicted or not, whether these battles resolve into consensus or not, whether scientific accounts yet find themselves embraced by those they describe or not. This observation could well have been made a decade ago, when one of the authors of this book, Helen Keane, published her first major work on the subject, *What's Wrong with Addiction?* (2002). Animated by a related interest in the meanings of addiction, that book tracked and systematically unpacked contemporary certitudes of drug and other addiction, opening up questions that we are still exploring and refining today. Importantly, however, the last decade has yielded a range of theoretical advances that aid us in thinking drugs and addiction afresh. Some of these inform the project this book undertakes and can be seen in various manifestations in other work on drugs that has emerged in recent years.

Situating a social science of addiction

In taking up this project, our book builds upon a long tradition of critical social science on drug use. Sociological and ethnographic studies have illuminated the meanings and practices of drug use in communities and cultures around the world, and this work constitutes an impressive corpus on which social scientists of addiction are wise to draw. However, the corpus of social science literature on addiction *per se* is nowhere near as developed. In a recent review, Darin Weinberg (2011) points out the contrast between the abundance of literature which provides detailed descriptions of drug cultures, drug use and drug users and the paucity of work specifically investigating addiction. As he states, naturalistic and ethnographic studies of drug use have been concerned with exploring the meanings of drug use as a social practice and experience and have therefore tended to avoid the moralised topic of addiction. The avoidance of addiction, however, cannot be solely understood as an intellectual and political squeamishness about moral judgement. The problem of addiction as a description of, or explanation for, behaviour from a sociological perspective is that it is almost inextricably linked to the medical and therapeutic discourse which dominates both the study of drug use and everyday thinking and talking about drugs. As well as ushering in a moralising framework, addiction too easily installs a perspective which places the individual pathologies of drug use at the centre of the picture – exactly the approach to drug use that the ethnographic impulse seeks to challenge.

Nevertheless, as Weinberg's review demonstrates, the sociology of addiction has expanded into a vibrant subfield marked by promising theoretical approaches. Early critical work reflected the origins of the category of addiction by focusing on alcohol and heroin dependence as the classic forms. Emerging neuroscientific models of addiction promote a view of addiction as a pathological relationship that can develop with a seemingly unlimited range of substances and activities. The scope of a recently published edited collection, *Critical Perspectives on Addiction* (Netherland 2012), speaks to the current interest in this changing landscape of addiction science and treatment.

In a section on the expansion of addiction, this text includes chapters on obesity and video gaming, two of the new additions to addiction discourse.

Importantly, however, one of these chapters, a historical analysis of self-help weight-loss programmes, actually challenges the idea that addiction has only recently expanded into these non-drug fields (Parr & Rasmussen 2012). It points out that the idea of addiction to food was circulating in both popular and medical discourse in the 1940s, albeit within a psychoanalytic rather than neuroscientific framework. This question about the usefulness and limitations of a trope of expansion in understanding the contemporary landscape of addiction is one we explore in this book. We wish to take the analysis beyond a simple additive pattern in which new substances and behaviours are brought into a stable and singular model of addiction. Rather, we aim to highlight the way the category of addiction itself is inevitably challenged and changed by the inclusion of new versions of compulsive attachment, as well as the way different addictions interact or fail to interact in this conceptual field. The value of such an approach is demonstrated in a chapter 'Critical Perspectives on Addiction' on the role of nicotine replacement therapy (NRT) in confirming the need for a model of addiction which incorporates desire in excess of dependence (Elam 2012).

Before reviewing recent texts and themes, however, it is important to acknowledge the existence of an influential tradition of critical scholarship on the concept of addiction. Central to this tradition are studies which reveal the way addiction as an explanatory concept based on 'the loss of control' becomes possible and meaningful only in particular historical and cultural locations (Levine 1978; Room 1985; Berridge 1999; Reinarman 2005). These social constructionist studies treated 'addiction' and 'the addict' as created and culture-bound categories rather than natural types, thereby questioning the medical and scientific project of identifying the universal truth of addiction.

In his classic article 'The Discovery of Addiction', Harry Levine argued that in 18th-century America drunkenness, even habitual drunkenness, was regarded as natural and normal. People were assumed to drink to excess because they wanted to, and because they loved alcohol. Levine (1978) argues that addiction as a disease of the will came to make sense only when self-control became a vital individual and social value with the rise of the middle class in the 19th century. In a body of work spanning four decades, Robin Room (1985, 1998, 2001, 2003) has developed this socio-historical approach into a detailed and multidimensional understanding of addiction as a concept and experience that is enmeshed with systems of globalisation, industrialisation and commercialisation. In his work, addiction as a disorder is a 'shifting kaleidoscope'; definitions and 'governing images' of addiction change according to social trends, political ideologies and governmental regulations and medical institutions and traditions (1998, 2001). Crucially, for the approach taken by this book, Room has also highlighted the 20th-century trend within the *DSM* towards an inclusive framing of addiction so that a concept originally developed to describe alcohol and opiate dependence became applicable across a range of very different psychoactive substances (1998).

The critical literature which has developed from this socio-cultural tradition has been deeply influenced by the work of Foucault and his understandings of the relationship between knowledge, power and subjectivity. The idea that addiction operates as a powerful therapeutic and political discourse which classifies, normalises and disciplines subjects has been a productive analytic tool in many studies (Valverde 1998; Bourgois 2000; Fraser & valentine 2008, Keane 2009). A recent ethnographic study which takes a semiotic approach to the experience of addiction treatment demonstrates the continuing value of apprehending 'the addicted subject' as a product of the structures set up to treat him or her. In her analysis of a US treatment programme for homeless women, E. Summerson Carr points out the remarkable emphasis the staff placed on language and on talking. She argues that the programme's aim of endowing people with 'lasting sobriety' and 'self-sufficiency' was primarily about reconfiguring the clients' relationship to language and training them in a particular way of speaking about the self (2011, 3). Carr (2011, 4) calls this prescribed mode of speaking 'the ideology of inner reference', an ideology which 'presumes that (1) "healthy" language refers to pre-existing phenomena, and (2) the phenomena to which it refers are internal to speakers'. The demand for 'honest' inner referentiality produces the clients' addicted subjectivity as fundamentally a problem of self-deception. It also acts to filter out their social commentary and institutional critiques.

Carr's work demonstrates that addiction as an entity internal to and confined within the self emerges from treatment rather than preceding it. Through a fine-grained linguistic analysis, she maps out the specific model of addicted subjectivity that the 'Fresh Beginnings' programme brings into being through staff–client interactions. This is a topographical model in which access to a 'storehouse' of inner truths is blocked by layers of shame, anger and denial, and therefore 'teaching clients to read and speak what they once denied and buried' is the primary goal of treatment (2011, 94). As we demonstrate in the following chapters, the kind of problem that addiction is depends on institutional location and the ontological politics of the substance involved. Self-knowledge and self-referentiality are not always so central.

Additional insight into the production of addicted subjectivity within specific treatment spaces is provided by recent studies of methadone maintenance treatment (MMT). The focus here is not primarily on language but on the social and spatial regulation of bodies (Bourgois 2000; Smith 2011). The requirement for daily attendance and the strict dosing schedules paradoxically produce MMT clients as dependent and inflexible subjects who struggle to manage work and family responsibilities (Fraser & valentine 2008). These effects of treatment are interpreted as symptoms of addiction and a drug-using lifestyle. Smith points out the particular articulations of addict identity fostered by the social and spatial segregation of MMT provision. In the Toronto clinic he studied, the space of the clinic and its exposed and highly surveilled location promoted stigmatisation and the inscription of users as non-productive and dangerous sources of contagion (2011, 299). As Fraser and valentine's Australian research demonstrates, the MMT clinic is made up of temporal as well as spatial arrangements. In the particular 'timespace' of MMT, addiction is a matter of waiting and queuing, often outside. This arrangement of bodies produces some of the unruliness and antisocial conduct which is again attributed to the internal qualities of addicts. Thus 'the chronotype of the clinic acts as much to produce particular kinds of clients as it does to treat them' (2008, 109).

Other recent work in this social constructionist tradition has analysed addiction more broadly as a concept that has gained new strength and salience in the context of neo-liberalism and late consumer capitalism. In contrast to earlier work which emphasised the importance of self-control to the ideal of the productive citizen, this work highlights the significance of consumption and freedom to contemporary norms of citizenship. Gerda Reith begins her Foucauldian genealogy of addiction by noting that in affluent societies consumption has become a prime site where individuals express values of freedom, autonomy, creativity and choice. In this context, addiction proliferates as a 'consumer pathology', a disorder which turns the 'sovereign consumer' on its head: 'transforming freedom into determinism and desire into need' (2004, 286). At a time when exercising free choice among a range of commodities is constitutive of identity, the notion of dependency takes on a 'particular horror'.

Toby Seddon (2010) has developed a similar argument about the enmeshment of addiction and understandings of freedom, although one more grounded in historical analysis of drug prohibition and regulation.

Seddon argues that liberal conceptions of freedom have been mutually constitutive of understandings of the problem of drugs as they developed in different phases over the past two centuries. He presents addiction as a capitalist concept, connected to the circulation of drugs as a global commodity. Thus transformations in capitalism can be linked to changes in the concept of addiction. The contemporary valorisation of consumerism co-exists with the idea of certain forms of disordered, repetitive consumption as a public menace.

Seddon and Reith's analyses share a Foucauldian perspective which is scouring of liberalism and attentive to large-scale transformations in regimes of power and knowledge. In Reith's account, addiction is a classic Foucauldian discourse, a mode of governance and control which acts through rather than against individual freedom. And although addiction in these accounts reflects the tensions and paradoxes of freedom in late modern societies, addiction discourse itself is presented as singular and unified in its character, structure and effects. One of Reith's key themes is the almost infinite ability of neo-liberal addiction discourse to produce new disordered identities such as pathological gamblers, bulimics, shopping addicts and Internet addicts. But while this expansionary process brings addiction into new areas of social life and into contact with different kinds of subjects, substances, activities and experiences, addiction itself remains fundamentally unchanged in its constitution of freedom and unfreedom. This monolithic effect is in part an inevitable result of Reith's ambitious (and valuable) attempt to outline a genealogy of addictive consumption in the space of one article. However, it also emerges from the Foucauldian framework which focuses on concepts of power, knowledge and authority and approaches medicine and the psy disciplines primarily as agents of regulation.

From this perspective, it is possible to interpret the 21st-century neuroscience of addiction as simply an updated and perhaps even more reductive and hubristic version of earlier discursive formations. While the brain disease model refers to neurotransmitters and reward systems rather than personality types or character flaws, it still operates to pathologise and regulate individuals and demonise certain forms of consumption. Against this critical impulse, Nikolas Rose (2007) has argued that neurochemical styles of thought in fact lift the moral weight associated with addiction, because they detach the disorder from the personality and character of the individual and refigure it as a correctible anomaly. Others see a more ambivalent mix of potential effects, including the increased stigma and social distancing that occurs when neurological 'others' are created (Buchman et al. 2010).

More importantly for our purposes, the rise of the brain disease model of addiction, and the increasing prominence of neuroscience more generally, has promoted a new engagement of critical addiction scholars with the biology of addiction and drugs. In 2006, Howard Kushner criticised historians of addiction (with some notable exceptions) for ignoring biology in their desire to highlight the cultural construction of addiction and its political and social meanings. He noted that when biology did appear in historical works, it was contrasted to, rather than integrated with, cultural understandings. For example, in one typical text, biology was treated as 'an essentialized undifferentiated trope, which requires no explanation or investigation' (2006, 137). Kushner (2010, 8) called for an interdisciplinary 'cultural biology of addiction' which could bring together 'seemingly contradictory social-constructionist and biologically reductionist claims about addictions'.

Kushner's challenge echoed the sustained and wide-ranging criticisms of social constructionist approaches to science which had emerged from feminist and science studies scholars. The essence of this criticism was that by giving the determining role in the construction of reality to language and culture, social science and humanities scholars have been unable to engage with materiality and have in fact divested the material of all agency and influence (Fraser & valentine 2008; Hekman 2010; Fraser & Seear 2011). The critical impulse which had set out to challenge positivism by reading science as a text had become a limiting orthodoxy, imposing unnecessary theoretical constraints on the field. As Bruno Latour (1993, 90) put it in his characteristically provocative style, 'Are you not fed up at finding yourself forever locked into language alone, or imprisoned in social representations alone, as so many social scientists would like you to be?'

This lack of attention to materiality not only produces attenuated versions of reality and limits the impact of socio-cultural critique but also reproduces dualisms of nature and culture, biology and society and human and non-human. As Kushner and others have noted, social science and humanities perspectives on addiction have until recently demonstrated the foreclosure of the biological characteristic of social constructionism. They have tended to assume either that there is no genuine biophysiological basis for addiction or that the biological basis is a fixed substrate for the regulatory discourse which is where the real interest and action lie (Vrecko 2010a).

In response to the limitations of traditional socio-cultural critique, critical scholars of addiction have in recent years turned their attention to some neglected core elements of addiction. The three elements we will discuss briefly here are

- the scientific and technical content of addiction science (other than as a form of ideology or mechanism of social control);
- the agency of substances and other material objects in the production of addiction; and
- the phenomenology of addiction, its emotional and embodied impact (other than as a discursively constructed form of subjectivity).

Our discussion is selective rather than comprehensive. We review key social science works that respond innovatively to each of these issues and open the terrain of critical addiction studies into a more materialist mode.

Addiction science

In her 2007 book *Discovering Addiction*, Nancy Campbell maps the social and scientific networks of US addiction research in the 20th century, showing how substance abuse researchers produced the science of addiction that has become part of our everyday thinking and talking about drugs. While Campbell focuses on the 'thought collectives' and 'epistemic communities' that formed in particular labs, her analysis also takes in the materiality, contingency and uncertainty of scientific research. As well as communities of scientists, the discovery of addiction was dependent on prison inmates and 'junkie monkeys' who were enrolled into the research enterprise in order to perform addiction and relapse. As Campbell (2007, 222) states, '"Addiction" evolved from the meandering interplay of multiple methods, subfields, experimental subjects, and objects of knowledge.' Despite their best efforts, the scientists involved were finally unable to stabilise one set of answers to the questions they asked about the nature of addiction; addiction remained stubbornly multiple. Campbell's book ends with the transformation of addiction research from a field dominated by behavioural pharmacology to the neuroscientific enterprise of the 21st century.

Within the sociological literature on the neuroscience of addiction, Scott Vrecko's analyses stand out for their nuanced examination of the 'addiction neuropolitics' that has enabled addiction to emerge as a disease of the brain. His work takes seriously the insights of addiction medicine and includes the biological components of the addiction experience. However, it also maintains a 'critical ambivalence towards the reality of addiction as a disease', arguing that the biomedical discourses themselves support this ambivalence (2010a, 38). Vrecko presents a detailed historicised account of how addiction was brought into being as a brain disease through an assembling of material, political and social forces. He begins by questioning what it means to state 'addiction is a brain disease' as an objective fact, as many authorities now do. Rather than taking a fact to be a transcendent and value-free truth, he draws on the work of philosopher of science Ludwig Fleck to examine the scientific facts of addiction as historical events that are brought into existence in concrete and specific contexts. This is not to deny facts their objective existence but to reveal the work that is done to produce and reproduce them (2010b).

In his account of the rise of post-war addiction science, Vrecko highlights the mutual enrolment between a small group of scientists interested in the neurobiology of addiction and agents in the US government who identified drug problems, especially heroin addiction, as a threat to social order and national security. Addiction scientists became players in a 'juridically willed research economy' in which generous funding enabled basic research to flourish (2010b, 58). This research included the identification of opiate receptors by a group of US scientists in the 1970s, an event recognised as a breakthrough in the establishment of addiction as a brain disease. But Vrecko points out that research on the 'receptor' pre-existed its actual 'discovery' because the existence of the receptor as a hypothetical entity was necessary for pharmacological theories to make sense. Thus experimental methods were developed to 'select, purify, filter and shape the physiological phenomena that came to be identified as receptors' (2010b, 61). Through this kind of assembling of political, practical, technical and material elements, addiction was formed as a disorder situated in 'the newly developing problem space' of the brain.

The value of this perspective is that it recognises the historical contingency of addiction science and the reliance of facts on technical, political and social support without denying or ignoring the existence of the biological. It allows Vrecko (2010a, 40) to argue that in the domain of medical science 'addiction used to be one thing and now it is something else'. Specifically, he argues that contemporary brain science has produced a new kind of 'drug-independent' addiction which includes behavioural problems such as gambling and shopping. This is not just a matter of discursive construction but the result of the actions of anti-craving medications such as naltrexone on the brains of affected individuals. This book shares a similar interest in the historical contingency of biological phenomena, and we develop our conceptual approach to the issue in later pages using tools drawn from the field of science and technology studies (STS).

The agency of substances

The question of how certain substances act to produce addiction has been central to addiction science, but until recently has not received much attention from social scientists. Pharmacological discourse classifies psychoactive 'drugs of abuse' as substances which have the ability to turn previously normal and autonomous individuals into 'addicts' because of their unique chemical properties (Keane 2002). Because social scientists have been committed to undermining this taken-for-granted chemical determinism, they have tended to analyse drugs primarily as a rhetorical and political category, created through legal regulation and medical knowledge and deployed in order to distinguish normal from abnormal consumption. But the shift to more materialist analyses has led critical addiction scholars to return to the question of substances and their effects, at the same time as addiction science is moving away from the view of addictiveness as a quality internal only to drugs. This has produced fertile ground for a general rethinking of questions of agency and causality in relation to addiction. What is it that drives particular addictive processes and how does the answer to this question influence the types of intervention deemed most appropriate and effective?

In the work of STS scholars such as Emilie Gomart, the materiality of substances is foregrounded but in a very different way from the pharmacological model of drugs as fixed and constant in their properties, fundamentally unchanged by the processes in which they are involved. Instead, substances are refigured as assemblages of effects that are brought into being or performed in particular experimental or clinical contests. Using the tools of actor network theory, Gomart (2002, 126) has examined the way heroin and methadone are performed in two different sets of experiments, one in France and one in the United States, highlighting the 'tentative constructions of differences' between the substances that occur in each case. Her point is that the effects of methadone (including its relationship to addiction) are not properties of the substance but are actions brought into being by networks of techniques, objects and actors. It is these effects which become temporarily stabilised into 'a substance' through the work done in the laboratory.

Similarly, in a study of opioid pharmacotherapy treatment at a French clinic, Gomart highlights the way methadone and other drugs were not fixed and deterministic in their impact on users, rather their actions emerged only when they were put into relation with specific techniques of use. Thus, in opioid pharmacotherapy treatment there is a reciprocal construction of user and drug: both substance and patient are empowered; they 'potentialise' each other (2004, 99). Significantly, this is empowerment through the application of constraints in order to achieve a more stable life. This understanding of addiction and its treatment questions both the dominant view of addiction as slavery and a critical account of addiction discourse as inevitably oppressive. Gomart demonstrates how freedom and dependence are put into a non-oppositional relationship in methadone treatment in that the phenomenon of addiction is included in the intervention. Methadone, an addictive substance, is part of the (re-)construction of the addict as a human subject but is effective only within a particular network of treatment and with particular kinds of clients.

The materiality of methadone is also foregrounded in Fraser and valentine's Australian study of MMT (mentioned earlier). One of their concerns is the traditional cultural studies topic of representation, specifically media accounts of methadone and their use of metaphor. In their analysis, representation is not simply about the production of meaning; it is rather inseparable from the ontology of methadone as a phenomenon in the world. In particular, the repeated designation of methadone as a replacement/substitute for heroin constitutes it as doubly marginalised (2008, 55). In being like heroin, methadone is dangerous, disorderly and addictive; but in being 'not heroin', it is inauthentic. These problematic attributes are not pre-existing qualities of the drug but formed as part of the materialisation of methadone.

As Fraser and valentine point out, a focus on materiality and the agency of objects enables a move beyond the obsession with individual human agency in accounts of drug use and addiction. If we think of addiction as a set of relations between human and non-human objects, techniques, locales and practices, it is no longer a pathology chained to a regulatory ideal of freedom of will. Addiction also becomes more variable, constituted as a different phenomenon depending on the form of consumption or behaviour that is the target of intervention. Like Gomart's discussion of opioid pharmacotherapy treatment, this work suggests new avenues for investigating 'drug effects' (Fraser & Moore 2011). Indeed, the analysis we conduct in this book aims to make use of these new avenues. Each chapter seeks to illuminate the ways different material objects of addiction (methamphetamine, alcohol and food) remake addiction as a phenomenon.

The posthumanist phenomenology of addiction

One of the complaints that can be made about critical addiction studies is that its commitment to social constructionism and to analysing addiction as a discourse has led to a lack of engagement with the embodied experience of addiction and the suffering it entails (Weinberg 2002, Bourgois & Schonberg 2009). An overemphasis on, for example, the totalising discourse of addiction found in Alcoholics Anonymous texts can obscure the powerful practical effects of everyday 12-step ethics on lives that have become unmanageable (Valverde & White-Mair 1999). In some cases, this demand for more emphasis on lived experience is symptomatic of a suspicion of or unfamiliarity with poststructuralist theory, and a desire to reinstall an unreflective humanism as the truth of drugs and addiction. Reifying the human as the source of all action and meaning is particularly problematic in relation to addiction discourse, which draws its power and influence in part from its invocation of the self as the site of disorder and health. In any case, a large and diverse ethnographic and qualitative literature exists on drug use, including addictive use, that does foreground first-person experience and the meanings of this experience to the individuals involved (Keane 2011). Critical addiction studies have value precisely because they supplement rather than replicate this literature on drug use. That said, Weinberg (2011) has recently argued convincingly that specifically *posthumanist* approaches to social research provide theoretical tools better equipped to understand the experience of addiction than the alternatives offered by humanism and social constructionism. For example, in the work of Gomart and Fraser and valentine (discussed earlier), addiction is presented along posthumanist lines as an assemblage of interacting entities (including humans, texts, substances, objects and technologies). Similarly, a 'lifetime of attachment to the syringe' as a feature of addicted subjectivity has recently been explored by Nicole Vitellone (2010), with an emphasis on the affective nature of this attachment.

Weinberg suggests that a posthumanist approach enables a uniquely productive way of reading the accounts of individuals suffering from addiction gathered in qualitative research. He is particularly concerned with developing a sociological understanding of the loss of control which is frequently and vividly described in such accounts. Because of its centrality to medical and moral models of addiction, critical scholars have tended to interpret the notion of 'loss of control' as a normalising mechanism, highlighting its inability to capture the social practices of drug users (Moore 1992; Room 2003). However, Weinberg argues that the functioning of self-control as a regulatory ideal does not mean that the experience of loss of control and the suffering it causes can be reduced to a construct or justificatory device. His point is that things other than human subjects can be the source of suffering, and addiction is often (but not inevitably) such a thing. He conceptualises addictions as 'non-human agents residing in the bodies of those who are addicted' (2011, 307). In contrast to most critical scholars, he emphasises the harm and alienation of addiction and identifies it as a disease, albeit through the use of a nuanced posthumanist definition. He argues that if we take diseases to be 'patterns of *harmful* [emphasis in original] bodily articulation', patterns 'with which we cannot, or do not want to, identify our selves...', then there is 'no reason to deny, and every reason to affirm, that an addiction might be just such a thing' (2011, 307).

This position is one we will revisit in various ways in the chapters that follow. The conceptualisation of addiction as an agent internal to the addict's body raises questions about the relationship between the inner space of the individual and the external space of 'the environment'. One of the characteristics of the brain disease model of addiction is a very thin understanding of 'the environment' or 'social context' as a distal and secondary factor which merely 'influences' the development of addiction in individuals (Campbell 2007; Vrecko 2010a). Refiguring the idea of environment and context seems crucial to us as the neuroscience of addiction continues to be developed and affirmed as the explanation for all problems of excessive consumption and attachment. In addition, we would argue that the idea of suffering itself needs to be carefully explored as a phenomenon which itself emerges from a network of elements and forces (Bourgois & Schonberg 2009). Another issue is the tendency in Weinberg's conceptualisation to tie addiction to a singular and negative affective register. Loss of control and suffering are not the only emotional and affective experiences reported in accounts of addiction (Vitellone 2010). Indeed, losing control can itself be a multiple phenomenon.

* * *

In summing up this overview of the critical social science literature on addiction, it is clear that the field has flourished in recent years, developing from an early focus on the culture-bound and historically specific nature of the 'disorder' to one that encompasses a promising range of theoretical approaches. Foucauldian perspectives treating addiction as a regulatory biopolitical discourse have remained important, but a new emphasis has emerged on the salience of addiction in the contemporary landscape of neo-liberalism and late consumer capitalism. In this context, the addict is a subject who fails to consume prudently and rationally, as well as one who has abandoned the ethics of productive citizenship. Other studies have focused on more specific manifestations of addiction, examining the way the disorder emerges from the structures and interventions devised to treat it rather than precede them. Here addiction becomes many different kinds of problems, rather than a singular phenomenon. Some forms of treatment prioritise spatial and temporal management of addicted subjects, while others focus on the development of self-knowledge and self-referentiality. Thus addiction varies not only according to the object of compulsive desire (whether legal substance, illicit drug or habitual behaviour) but according to the treatment response.

Finally, critical addiction studies are now characterised by a new interest in materiality and less overwhelmingly sceptical engagement with scientific discourses. Neurobiological phenomena and the particular agency of addictive substances have become incorporated into social and cultural analysis. This work has often involved the productive taking up of the insights of STS, an approach we draw on in this book (discussed in more detail below). As well as enabling a fuller account of the political, practical, technical and material elements which make up addiction, this posthumanist approach allows for a fresh understanding of the embodied experience of addiction.

Many valuable theoretical directions suggest themselves in the literature discussed here, and indeed some of our past works have already drawn on aspects of the literature cited so far (see, for example, Fraser 2006; Fraser & valentine 2008; Keane et al. 2011; Fraser & Moore 2011; Fraser & Seear 2011). Of especial relevance to the project we undertake in this book – tracing the shifting trajectories of addiction concepts across three areas (the methamphetamine 'crisis', alcohol addiction and the rise of binge drinking, and food addiction and obesity) – are four issues raised in the literature reviewed here. The first is the question of materiality posed in different ways by Gomart, Vrecko and Weinberg. The second is the importance of conceiving addiction, as does Campbell, as theoretically and practically multiple. The third is the need to reconsider reductive notions of 'environment' and their tendency to pre-empt the shape and boundaries of the research object of addiction itself, and the fourth is the need to keep in sight the importance of embodied experience as well as discursive formations.

In attending to the last issue identified above, we structure our book around two main bodies of data: 'expert' discourse (epidemiological, neuroscientific, public health and policy literatures) and 'public' discourse (interviews with people who fall into key public health target groups associated with each of the addiction areas we explore – methamphetamine consumers, young drinkers and mothers exposed to obesity-prevention education). By exploring changing definitions and understandings of addiction across these discursive domains, we are able to track the reach and shape of particular emerging ideas, their assumptions and implications, and the extent to which expertise informs the outlook of individuals who might be the objects of this expertise. In the process, we find significant disjunctions between the two, as well as within each. We also find important insights in the public discourse to which, we argue, the makers of expert knowledges ought more closely attend.

Before we proceed with our analysis, it is important to discuss in more detail the conceptual approach we take in the book. As the literature discussed already makes clear, the concepts we use have the potential to remake our objects of study in radically different ways, and as such there is little room for imprecision or inattention. To begin this discussion we turn to the work of STS scholar John Law, finding within it tools of particular keenness for the tasks we have set ourselves: to map and analyse the shifting phenomenon of contemporary addiction and to do so in ways that acknowledge the importance of *both* language and materiality – of reality as durable *and* emergent, as stable *and* multiple – of discourse and experience. These questions we ask about drugs and addiction require a critical approach to scientific knowledge. As we have noted, knowledge production on drugs, drug use and addiction has been largely dominated by the sciences, and it is on this scientifically defined knowledge that policies and strategies for acting on drug use have been based. Indeed, as we have argued elsewhere (Fraser & Moore 2011), an influential trend in recent approaches to drug policy has been the call for 'evidence-based policy', that is, policy developed not, it is argued, via 'moralising' approaches to drugs but through what advocates see as the 'objective', unbiased findings of scientific research (Wood 2010). While this approach has several strategic benefits, it also has weaknesses: (1) its tendency to take for granted that value-free, objective knowledge *can* be produced about the world, and (2) its active role in erasing the action of the sciences themselves in making the object to be studied – the object about which 'evidence' is to be collected. Among critical social scientists, this approach is challenged through a range of constructionist perspectives that expressly query the idea that the world pre-exists our attempts to know it. As we explain, this book takes inspiration from some of the most influential of these perspectives, drawing on STS to analyse addiction as a constructed 'social problem', and in doing so to rethink it, and its effects, in terms of new theories of reality.

Approach: Practices all the way down

What is addiction and on what are our fears about it based? What is the body, what is the brain? How do they function symbolically? What about drugs? Are they just chemicals, or do their meanings run deeper and resonate more widely than this? Clearly, addiction, bodies and drugs are not simple objects and should not be treated as such. This is no foundationalist claim. The character and attributes of these phenomena are not given in nature but *made in practice*, as John Law (2011), among others, might put it. They are made and made again in the meanings that accrue to them, that circulate through them, as they are enacted. In taking this approach to objects, we draw on John Law's recently published chapter 'Collateral realities' in Baert and Rubio's edited collection, *The Politics of Knowledge* (2011). In his chapter, Law conducts a close analysis of a presentation delivered to a conference on a topic quite different from that covered here: animal welfare. The presentation describes a large research project on farm animal welfare in the European Union (the conference was entitled 'Welfare Quality'). Specifically, Law analyses the PowerPoint slide show that accompanied the presentation, examining each slide for the 'collateral realities' it produces.

Law's notion of collateral realities is embedded in a theoretical framework highly relevant to this book's central concerns and which we have described elsewhere (see, for example, Fraser & Seear 2011). In brief, Law locates his work in an area sometimes called 'ontics' or 'ontological politics'. These terms refer to an approach to knowledge and materiality that owes much to social constructionism but takes an extra crucial step beyond some of its key features. Social constructionism contends that reality, including material objects and the 'natural world', is constituted by discourse and does not pre-exist society and culture (Goode & Ben-Yehuda 1994). This approach to reality has been embraced by scholars and others interested in transformational politics. If reality – even the natural world and material objects otherwise seen as immutable and given – is the product of discourse and the operations of social and cultural forces, the rationale goes, it cannot be used to justify existing social or political relations, existing social or political inequities and injustices. But while constructionism recognises the 'made-ness' of apparently given things such as diseases, it tends, according to the ontological politics approach taken by Law, to frame the process of this making as singular and terminal. That is, the making of a thing happens once, comes to an end and results in a stable object constituted in a certain way – a product of its social and temporal context to be sure, but complete and now immutable in its constructedness. As Annemarie Mol, one of John Law's (1999, 76) most frequent collaborators, puts it:

> Constructivist stories suggest that alternative 'constructions of reality' might have been possible. They have been possible in the past, but vanished before they ever fully blossomed.

Mol argues that, on the contrary, phenomena are always being made and remade – multiple processes of constitution occur over time and at any given time, shaped and informed by the various discourses in which they are inserted or from which they emerge. For Mol, this claim that realities are constantly in the making, and that the moment of construction is never complete or behind us, underwrites the political purchase of her research. This theoretical approach to reality has informed an impressive range and volume of scholarly research projects, including our own (for example, Fraser & valentine 2008; Fraser 2011; Fraser & Moore 2011; Fraser & Seear 2011; Keane et al. 2011; Moore 2011). In this book we focus on a specific tool that has emerged recently from this framework – that of collateral realities – as well as a more familiar concept from this field of theorising: the assemblage.

Analysing the assumptions at work in the slides accompanying the Welfare Quality presentation, Law argues that many 'collateral realities' are made in the process of enacting the central object of the presentation (the aforementioned research project). As he explains (2011, 156), collateral realities are

> realities that get done incidentally, and along the way. They are realities that get done, for the most part, unintentionally. They are realities that may be obnoxious. Importantly, they are realities could be different. It follows that they are realities that are through and through political.

Distinguishing the 'reality' intended in the expression 'collateral realities' from conventional accounts of reality, Law (2011, 156) points out:

> If reality *appears* (as it usually does) to be independent, prior, definite, singular or coherent then this is because it is being *done* that way [emphasis in the original]. Indeed these attributes or assumptions become examples, amongst others, of collateral realities.

In short, reality is not given, or even 'socially constructed' in the common sense, rather it is, as already suggested, 'done in *practice*'. As such it must be done and redone again to remain stable, is multiple, and very much open to change.

Law's interest in collateral realities, and in the general multiplicity and mutability of reality, is expressly empirical. When he describes realities as made in practice, he assumes along with this formulation the need to investigate these practices empirically (2011, 157) if we are to understand properly realities as they are made, and as they might be made differently. Practices, he says, are assemblages of relations. These assemblages can be mapped and tracked to yield knowledge about specific realities. As he puts it, 'We cannot work "in general", because there is no "in general" ' (2011, 157). There are only singular, unstable assemblages. The notion of the assemblage on which Law draws here owes much to the work of two theorists, Gilles Deleuze and Bruno Latour. As Deleuze has asserted (Deleuze & Parnet 2002, 51), 'The minimum real unit is not the word, the idea, the concept, or the signifier, but the assemblage.' What is this assemblage that forms the ontological basis of reality? Law cites Watson-Verran and Turnbull (2011, 157) here:

> [It's] like an episteme with technologies added but that connotes the ad hoc contingency of a collage in its capacity to embrace a wide variety of incompatible components. It also has the virtue of connoting active and evolving practices rather than a passive and static structure.

So the assemblage can be seen as an ad hoc cluster of knowledges, technologies, bodies and practices that contingently gather to form a temporary phenomenon, be it abstract or material. The world is made up of such assemblages, not of stable natural objects or self-evident, foundational concepts. One of these assemblages, we can surmise, is addiction.

To return to the notion of collateral realities, and Law's (2011, 158) example of the Welfare Quality conference presentation, he argues that the conference can be read as a moment of 'ontological politics'.

By this he means it constituted an occasion in which realities were being 'done' – both conventional and new, both explicitly concerned with animals and their welfare, and with a range of other issues 'collateral to' this central concern (2011, 161). The conference presentations and slide shows are not merely representations of reality, rather they enact it. It follows from this, then, that

> [i]f, performatively, representations do realities in practice, then those realities might have been done differently. We find ourselves in the realm of politics.

Law's approach to the particular presentation slide show he critiques corresponds with the approach to addiction we take in this book. Rather than merely reflecting a pre-existing reality, the texts and interviews we examine do ontological politics. They make realities, including, or partly through, collateral realities. Law (2011, 165) spells out the three main lessons he draws from treating the slide show he analyses in this way. First, it allows him to track very specifically the features of the enactments they undertake. How, precisely, do they work? By, he says, deploring textual strategies (here he cites selecting, juxtaposing, deleting and ranking elements). Second, these realities are not stable or consistent. Instead, different realities are enacted at different moments according to different needs. Third, he speculates that the multiplicity evident in the enacted realities he observes is a requirement of 'institutional survival' (2011, 165). Here he re-emphasises ontological politics and the role of collateral realities by adding that

> if this performative way of thinking shows that reals are done in multiple ways, then it also suggests that at least in principle those realities – or the balance between them – could be different.

In making this point Law also reminds us that realities should not be seen as the foundation for practices, or reflected in or revealed by practices. Rather, reality is 'practices all the way down' (2011, 165).

To clarify how this approach can be used across different empirical contexts, Law (2011, 171) suggests attention be paid to five related issues: first, consider how practices do realities, how relations are put together in particular order to 'produce objects, subjects and appropriate locations'; second, consider how these assemblages then become and remain stable. Third, identify the work being done 'to wash away the practices and turn representations into windows on the world' (2011,

171). How, in other words, do the processes through which realities are made and kept stable become sufficiently obscured to allow those realities to appear independent and anterior to the social? Fourth, remember that, whatever the empirical setting (he cites meeting halls, laboratories and surveys), there 'is no escape from practices' (2011, 171). In other words, all is practice; no other (founding) reality lurks behind them. Last, attend to 'gaps, aporias and tensions between the practices and their realities'. This is where the stability of realities can become vulnerable.

There is much to take from this approach in thinking addiction and, more specifically, in analysing the documents and interviews collected here for this purpose. Increasingly dominated by a neuroscientific account of addiction as brain disease and behaviour as the direct effect of brain chemistry, drug use and addiction are being 'done' in specific ways, constituted in part by (collateral) realities of the body, substance, nature and the social. In this book we consider the relations at work to constitute particular realities of addiction, how the stability of these realities is achieved and maintained, and the processes or strategies by which this stabilising work is simultaneously obscured or 'washed away' (Law 2011, 171). Are there gaps and tensions within the neuroscientific account and between it and public accounts of addiction? If so, how do these shape the realities enacted? In all these questions the role of collateral realities is, following Law, crucial. In his view (2011, 172), 'it is the endless enactment of collateral realities that tends to hold things steady'. We would add that, where critique is warranted, one or more of the collateral realities holding a particular reality stable may offer a useful entry point, that is, may prove vulnerable to destabilisation. In turn, other, related realities may be destabilised. As Law (2011, 174) reminds us:

> [W]hatever is not contested and, more particularly, whatever lies *beyond the limits of contestability* is that which operates most powerfully to do the real. And it is this, to be sure, that is the technique that lies at the heart of common sense realism. It is the enactment of collateral realities that turns what is being done in practice into what necessarily *has* to be [emphasis in the original].

In this book we go about examining discourses and practices of addiction that are at present going largely uncontested. We also look at discourses and practices of addiction that are attracting significant levels of contestation, consider the effects of this contestation and, most importantly, explore those elements within the debates that remain, despite much discussion and criticism, beyond the limits of contestability.

Consuming habits, making realities

One further point can be made here about the ontological approach to reality, and thus to addiction, we take up here. As becomes clear in the pages that follow, addiction is conceived in different ways by different interlocutors, but a theme that arises again and again among public accounts of addiction, that is, among those whose selves and lives have in some way or another directly encountered assemblages of addiction, is that of *habit*. Inspired by Eve Sedgwick's (1993) formative comments on the 'epidemic' of addiction attribution underway in the West, we find habit a promising direction for thinking about addiction.

Habits are, of course, as helpful as they are harmful. The *Oxford English Dictionary* (online version, accessed 8 July 2012) defines habit in many ways – its links with habitation, habitat and attire (especially the monk or nun's habit) are some obvious connections – but the opening definition is:

> a settled or regular tendency or practice, especially one that is hard to give up:
>
> - *he has an annoying habit of interrupting me*
> - *good eating habits*

As such, habit is neither good nor bad. As Sedgwick (1993, 138) puts it, offering habit as an 'otherwise' to the unforgivingly polarising, naively normalising, contemporary reflex of addiction attribution, habit is

> not opposed to [addiction] or explanatory of it, but rather one step to the side of it…a version of repeated action that moves, not towards metaphysical absolutes [of absolute voluntarity or absolute compulsion], but toward interrelations of the action – and the self acting – with the bodily habitus, the apparelling habit, the sheltering habitation, everything that marks the traces of that habit on a world that the metaphysical absolutes would have left in a vacuum.

The connections with Latour and Law's ontologies of the assemblage and realities are not hard to draw out here. Indeed, Sedgwick's conceptual embeddness in the exceptionally fertile poststructuralist field of queer theory (and its own rejection of foundationalist, stable subjects, objects and identities) means that her take on habit offers something unique to a debate that was already playing out around the meaning and value of habit in 20th-century philosophy, and which has found its way into some scholarly accounts of addiction. Mariana Valverde's (1998) classic work on alcoholism is a key example here. In exploring changing definitions of alcoholism over two centuries, her book also tracks the rise and fall of ideas of habit throughout this history. Valverde contextualises this discussion in American pragmatist philosophy, and particularly the work of William James, Charles Pierce and John Dewey, pointing to the way in which habit has been understood through various binaries such as free will versus natural necessity, with habit seen as the opposite of volition. As Valverde (1998, 38) explains, Dewey argued that the long-standing denigration of habit in Western philosophy and culture is based in the myth of the transcendental subject. She identifies precursors to Michel Foucault's arguments in his approach, observing, 'Dewey notes that "the doctrine of a single, simple and indissoluble soul was the cause and effect of the failure to recognise that concrete habits are the means of knowledge and thought"' rather than an obstacle to them. Valverde's book does not refer to Sedgwick's piece, but the scope to make links is clear. Sedgwick too works from a place of scepticism about the transcendental subject (one which is, of course, also precluded in Latour and Law's posthumanist ontology of the assemblage). She too sees habit as able, if only it is allowed, to exceed the many binaries attendant upon the narrow oppositional accounts of free will and determinism that so readily shape judgements about drug use. But mobilising habit in this different way is no easy task, she warns:

> It is extraordinarily difficult to imagine an analytically usable language of habit, in a conceptual landscape so rubbled and defeatured by the twin hurricanes named Just Do It and Just Say No.

While we would agree with this caution, we cannot resist but to try for such a language, offering an encounter between assemblages, collateral realities and habit to do so. What are realities, if we are to accept them as multiply made and remade, performed and enacted, dependent upon repetition for stability, for their very existence, if not habits? This is no idle speculation. If accepted, it would mean a fundamental shift in the status of habit from at best a way of modulating or refining reality, at worst of diminishing or obscuring it, to that of reality's very foundation.

Could it be, in other words, that addiction (as habit) might form the template for an ontological politics of reality?

This book is in some ways an experiment in this conjecture. We see addiction as assemblage, made and remade in different ways in discourse and the collateral realities it enacts to stabilise its specific materialisations. These enactments are also habits – and while we take in habit's implication of repetition here, we also recognise that repetition always risks (and is the prerequisite for) change. Elsewhere (Fraser & valentine 2008), having analysed the denigration of MMT as mere stasis, we attempted to recuperate repetition from its association with stagnation and unoriginality. Following feminists suspicious of the links commonly drawn between repetition, reproduction, stasis and femininity (Deutscher 2006, after Butler 1990), we argued that repetition entails rupture as much as stability. Now we wish (unapologetically) to *revisit* this idea. Ultimately our aim throughout this book is to map the ways in which contemporary enactments of addiction are remaking its meanings, and to invite in the process new considerations of habit and its uses for thinking consumption and compulsion.

Structure of the book

The book is organised into four parts. The first part (Chapter 1) details the two main fields and processes of expert knowledge production currently shaping concepts of addiction: neuroscientific research and the negotiations over the recently released fifth edition of the *DSM*. The second part moves into our first specific area of investigation, which focuses on the rise of concern about methamphetamine use. It is composed of two chapters. In the first of these (Chapter 2) we examine influential research texts to consider how claims about methamphetamine consumption are remaking addiction in new ways. In the second (Chapter 3) we consider how closely these remade addictions are re-enacted in policies aimed at addressing methamphetamine use, and in the ways individuals described in research and addressed by policies talk about their own consumption practices and bodily experiences of drug use. How much agreement can be found between the ways research, policy and affected individuals articulate methamphetamine consumption and addiction?

The third part of the book follows a similar structure to the second, this time taking alcohol as its focus. In the first of two chapters (Chapter 4), we take a close look at the controversy over alcohol addiction (or dependence) that has marked research and policy on drinking over the last 40 years. Despite occupying a central place in addiction discourse, alcohol dependence has proven very difficult to stabilise for experts. How do drinkers understand alcohol addiction or dependence? This is the focus of the following chapter (Chapter 5), in which we consider how closely expert notions of alcohol addiction mesh with everyday drinking practices, using interviews conducted with young drinkers – a key target group for public health injunctions against excessive alcohol consumption.

In the last of the book's four parts, this structure is followed again. The first of two chapters (Chapter 6) covers expert territory, this time examining scientific research on a new area of addiction attribution: obesity. Reflecting the growing influence of addiction frameworks in scientific discussions of overeating, we find expert discourse focusing with increasing energy on obesity as a symptom of food addiction, and neuroscience as the primary discipline for understanding food addiction. In the final chapter (Chapter 7) we draw on interviews with women whose role as mothers exposes them to a range of obesity-prevention discourses. As in the previous sections, these interviews allow us to reflect upon the extent to which expert accounts of substances and their effects have gained currency in public contexts – how well they articulate everyday experiences of consumption, how closely they reflect individual understandings of the relationship between drugs, bodies and daily lives, and how much space remains between accounts for introducing new queries, debates and habits of thought and practice.

The book's Conclusion draws together the findings from each of the sections, using new theory from Steve Woolgar and Bruno Latour to speculate further on the remaking of drugs in addiction discourses, and, in turn, the remaking of addiction in the politics of science, health and everyday life.

1
Models of Addiction

The use of psychoactive substances in order to alter mood or consciousness, alleviate suffering, improve performance or enhance social relations is characteristic of human cultures. For some individuals, the use of these substances becomes a pattern of habitual and persistent consumption that results in negative physical, emotional, relational and social effects. The range and intensity of these harmful effects is highly varied, depending on the specific substance and the context of use. Frequently, the harms of consumption co-occur with benefits. For example, smokers face the serious health risks and physical problems caused by cigarettes, but may also experience positive effects of relaxation, productivity and sociability. And because nicotine consumption is not generally said to cause intoxication and is a legal although highly regulated practice, tobacco dependence is quite different from illicit drug use and heavy drinking in its social meanings and effects.

Addiction can be understood as a culturally and historically specific set of ideas and practices that shapes the varied problems and predicaments of alcohol and other drug use into a singular and somewhat abstract entity: a disorder of compulsion located in the individual. This, in turn, promotes particular ways of thinking about selfhood. As Kane Race (2009, 15) puts it, addiction produces the self as the moral locus of consumption. But addiction is more than just a concept or field of knowledge; it is a practice, in that it is something that is *done* in specific contexts. To use the framework of ontological politics developed by John Law and Annemarie Mol in various works (see, for example, Mol 1999; Law 2011), the reality of addiction is brought into being in research labs, clinical encounters, health policy meetings, legal schedules and texts such as the *DSM*. Addiction is produced in these contexts through the assemblage of certain elements and the exclusion of others.

An object of study or target of intervention is stabilised out of the messy, fluid and heterogeneous social worlds of drug use and drug users (see Moore 1992), and various collateral realities are produced along the way.

As with many forms of human behaviour, medical and scientific discourse has become the most influential and authoritative source of knowledge about addiction. Scientific knowledge about addiction is a particularly powerful version of ontological politics because it is 'believed to reveal the inner workings of brains, minds, and bodies' (Campbell 2007, 1). It stabilises addiction as an objectively verifiable disorder or disease and employs terms such as 'symptom', 'pathology', 'natural history' and 'relapse' to reinforce the medical nature of drug-related experiences. As we show in this book, science valorises the development of a unified and universally applicable account of the nature of compulsive drug use as the goal of addiction research, and constitutes this form of knowledge as the key to solving the problem of drug use.

As an entity which implies the need for some sort of therapeutic intervention, addiction is also enacted as a technology of government. It promotes action on the conduct of others or the conduct of the self, in order to fashion a form of ethical subjectivity based on prudential consumption and responsible citizenship (Valverde 1998; Fraser & valentine 2008). The government of addiction takes many different forms, from court-ordered treatment to the open-ended work on the self fostered by 12-step groups. It can involve the provision of substitute drugs to manage dependence (as in the case of MMT or NRT) or the withdrawal of access to drugs (as can happen to pain patients on opiate therapy who develop 'aberrant' drug-seeking behaviour) (Keane & Hamill 2010). The aim may be for the drug user to internalise particular codes of conduct and beliefs about the self, or the goal may be a much more localised shift in appetitive behaviour. It is not just that the kinds of treatment that make sense depend on how addiction is defined; it is that the treatment technique itself constitutes and stabilises the problem of addiction (Bacchi 2009).

The government of addiction as a regulatory project is not simply about self-improvement. It cannot be separated from understandings of drug use, especially illicit drug use, as a pernicious and recalcitrant legal, social and moral problem. The disorder of addiction is not just destructive of the self; it is seen as a threat to social order, family life and the well-being of the nation. As agents of addiction, drugs are themselves enacted as a category of particularly powerful and malevolent substances which are outside normal human existence (despite the historical and cultural ubiquity of their use). This is especially the case when the drug in question is viewed as alien and/or unnatural (Manderson 2011). Therefore, medical models of addiction inevitably interact with policies focused on the control of drug supply and the punishment of offenders. For example, the idea of the addict as an individual who suffers from diminished control over her or his actions can be mobilised to justify coerced treatment as a supplement to, or substitute for, imprisonment.

Currently, the dominant scientific paradigm is of addiction as a 'chronic relapsing brain disease' caused by drug-induced dysfunction in neurochemical reward systems. Advocates of the brain disease model assert that it will undermine moralised and punitive beliefs about addiction and usher in an era of enlightened policy responses and treatment (National Institute on Drug Abuse 2007). Medical models of addiction are often contrasted with moralistic perspectives in this way. But as we suggest in this chapter, medical models are themselves hybrid medical-ethical assemblages, built on culturally specific ideals such as self-control and autonomy and inevitably involving normative judgements about how to live and how to prioritise pleasures. And while the narrative of scientific progress presents the most recent models as replacing superseded and outmoded knowledge, elements of these earlier governing discourses remain in circulation (Room 2001).

So far, we have discussed addiction as if it is a problem restricted to the consumption of psychoactive substances. It is certainly the case that medical concern about addiction has focused on alcohol and other drugs, and the first medical models of addiction that developed in the 18th and 19th centuries were based on problems of heavy drinking and opiate use (Levine 1978; Berridge 1999). However, as our discussions of the *DSM* in this chapter, binge drinking in Chapter 2 and overeating and obesity in Chapter 6 demonstrate, addiction science and medicine are currently in an expansionary mode in relation to the scope of addiction. Forms of habitual behaviour previously excluded from the frame of genuine addiction because they did not involve psychoactive substances are now being incorporated through the enrolment of neuroscientific explanations. Compulsive patterns of gambling, internet use, eating, sex and shopping are understood to involve the same neural substrate as drug use. This expansion in the potential agents of addiction is significant in part because addiction designates more than a dysfunctional pattern of behaviour. In both medical and popular discourses it produces an identity, a type of person – the addict – who is defined in terms of pathological desires. Characterised as lacking control over their consumption, their behaviour and their lives, addicted subjects have been easily read as 'other' to the ideal of the rational, autonomous and self-regulating individual (Fraser 2006; Moore & Fraser 2006). The effect of this expansionary mode on the marginalised and stigmatised identity of 'addict' remains an open question. Some recent prevalence research suggests that where addiction is defined as an intense preoccupation with a behaviour that produces negative consequences, it becomes a problem of the majority rather than a minority. Does this mean that addiction should be understood not as an aberration but as 'a natural state of affairs as a human being' (Sussman et al. 2011, 46)?

In this chapter we critically examine two influential contemporary models of addiction: the mental disorder identified in the *DSM* of the American Psychiatric Association (APA) and, more briefly, the already-mentioned brain disease model. The chapter begins with a general discussion of the *DSM* and its constitution of substance-related disorders. This is followed by three sections which examine different aspects of the *DSM-5*[1]: (1) its model of Substance Use Disorder (SUD); (2) its redefining of addiction to include non-substance-related disorders; (3) the commentary and criticism that followed its publication. These three sections necessarily refer to the brain disease model of addiction as neuroscience was invoked both as a justification for changes to the *DSM* and as a reason to question its scientific validity. A more systematic and detailed critique of addiction neuroscience and the brain disease model is presented in the final two sections of the chapter.

While both *DSM* and brain disease models have the institutional and epistemological authority of medicine and science, they are the product of distinct histories and as such have different purposes. They thus bring into being different realities and different types of problem. The *DSM* model was developed as a diagnostic tool and is based on a list of observable or reportable symptoms. It is a category embedded in a system of nosological classification. It reflects a clinical tradition of thinking about addiction in relation to harm, as well as contemporary psychiatry's demand for operationalisation. However, its influence goes far beyond the clinical as it provides the standard definition of addiction used in medical, epidemiological and psychological research.[2] Thus when psychopharmacologists study the effect of a certain treatment on cocaine addicts, the research subjects have usually qualified as addicts through the application of the *DSM* criteria. Or when epidemiologists study the prevalence of alcohol dependence on college campuses, they use the *DSM* criteria to determine who is counted in this category.

The fifth edition of the *DSM*, the *DSM-5*, was published in May 2013. It is the first new edition of the manual in two decades and its creation was a 'massive undertaking' which, according to the APA, involved evaluating all the diagnostic criteria and considering every aspect of the manual's organisation (APA 2013a, 5). Thirteen expert work groups undertook the task of proposing revisions, including a group devoted to substance-related disorders headed by Charles O'Brien. O'Brien is one of the most prominent addiction researchers in the United States, whose work encompasses the neurobiological and clinical aspects of addiction, including pharmacotherapy. A draft of the new manual was released in 2010 for professional and public comment, and 13,000 responses were received via the dedicated website (APA 2013a, 8). The final version of the *DSM-5* contains significant changes to several categories of disorder, including those related to substance use, as well as some important organisational changes. However, there is also a great deal of continuity between *DSM-5* and *DSM-IV*.

Unlike the *DSM*, the brain disease model is a causal explanation rather than a list of symptoms designed for clinical use. Although it stabilises addiction as an organic and observable neurobiological condition, it cannot be used to determine who is or is not addicted in the way the *DSM* can. It is a product of technoscientific research and offers a neurochemical and molecular account of the underlying process that produces the disordered behaviour of the addict. This is not to suggest that there are no connections or interactions between the models and the styles of thought they represent. One of the stated aims of the *DSM-5* revision was the incorporation of new knowledge from neuroscience, brain imaging and genetics into psychiatric nosology. As we will see, however, this aim has remained largely unfulfilled.

One shared feature of the two approaches is an attempt to produce a generic and generalisable model applicable whatever the substance, its effects, its legal and social status or route of administration. In the *DSM-IV*, the seven diagnostic criteria of substance dependence (see Table 1.1) were applicable to the self-administration of any 'class of substances except caffeine'. The manual also stated that 'the symptoms of dependence are similar across the various categories of substances', although it is noted that some symptoms are less salient for some classes of drugs and in a few instances not all of the symptoms are applicable (APA 2000, 192).

In the *DSM-5*, 11 diagnostic criteria make up the general model of 'substance use disorder', although not all are applied to every class of drug. Table 1.2 shows these 11 criteria as they appear in the specific diagnostic category opioid use disorder. The production of a general

Table 1.1 *DSM-IV* substance dependence criteria

A. A maladaptive pattern of substance use, leading to clinically significant impairment or distress, as manifested by three (or more) of the following, occurring at any time in the same 12-month period:

1) Tolerance, as defined by either of the following:
    a) A need for markedly increased amounts of the substance to achieve intoxication or desired effect
    b) Markedly diminished effect with continued use of the same amount of the substance
2) Withdrawal, as manifested by either of the following:
    a) The characteristic withdrawal syndrome for the substance (refer to Criteria A and B of the criteria sets for withdrawal from the specific substances)
    b) The same (or a closely related) substance is taken to relieve or avoid withdrawal symptoms
3) The substance is often taken in larger amounts or over a longer period than was intended.
4) There is a persistent desire or unsuccessful efforts to cut down or control substance use.
5) A great deal of time is spent in activities necessary to obtain the substance (e.g., visiting multiple doctors or driving long distances), use the substance (e.g., chain-smoking), or recover from its effects.
6) Important social, occupational, or recreational activities are given up or reduced because of substance use.
7) The substance use is continued despite knowledge of having a persistent or recurrent physical or psychological problem that is likely to have been caused or exacerbated by the substance (e.g., current cocaine use despite recognition of cocaine-induced depression, or continued drinking despite recognition that an ulcer was made worse by alcohol consumption).

Source: Reprinted with permission from the Diagnostic and Statistical Manual of Mental Disorders, Fourth Edition, Text Revision (Copyright © 2000). American Psychiatric Association.

category of addiction requires that differences between substances, such as the absence of withdrawal with hallucinogens and inhalants, are classified as exceptions to a general rule (APA 2013a, 483). It also rests on the generic nature of symptoms listed in the *DSM*, for example, 'the individual may spend a great deal of time obtaining the substance, using the substance or recovering from its effects' (2013a, 197). This is not a single symptom but rather a cluster of experiences

Table 1.2 *DSM-5* opioid use disorder criteria

A. A problematic pattern of opioid use leading to clinically significant impairment or distress, as manifested by at least two of the following, occurring within a 12-month period:

1) Opioids are often taken in larger amounts or over a longer period than was intended.
2) There is a persistent desire or unsuccessful efforts to cut down or control opioid use.
3) A great deal of time is spent in activities necessary to obtain the opioid, use the opioid, or recover from its effects.
4) Craving or a strong desire or urge to use opiods.
5) Recurrent opiod use resulting in a failure to fulfill major role obligations at work, school, or home.
6) Continued opioid use despite having persistent or recurrent social or interpersonal problems caused or exacerbated by the effects of opioids.
7) Important social, occupational, or recreational activities are given up or reduced because of opioid use.
8) Recurrent opioid use in situations in which it is physically hazardous.
9) Continued opioid use despite knowledge of having a persistent or recurrent physical or psychological problem that is likely to have been caused or exacerbated by the substance.
10) Tolerance, as defined by either of the following:

    a. A need for markedly increased amounts of opioids to achieve intoxication or desired effect.
    b. A markedly diminished effect with continued use of the same amount of the opioid.

Note: This criterion is not considered to be met for those taking opioids solely under appropriate medical supervision.

11) Withdrawal, as manifested by either of the following:

    a. The characteristic opioid withdrawal syndrome (refer to Criteria A and B of the criteria set for opioid withdrawal).
    b. Opioids (or a closely related) substance are taken to relieve or avoid withdrawal symptoms.

Note: This criterion is not considered to be met for those individuals taking opioids solely under appropriate medical supervision.

Source: Reprinted with permission from the Diagnostic and Statistical Manual of Mental Disorders, Fifth Edition, (Copyright © 2013). American Psychiatric Association.

related to time and its use. Presenting these different experiences as a single criterion allows behaviours as disparate as 'visiting multiple doctors or driving long distances' and 'chain-smoking' to be examples of the same symptom.

In the case of the brain disease model, whatever the subjective effects of different 'drugs of abuse', they are hypothesised to occur through the action of the neurotransmitter dopamine on a common neural pathway. This generalising approach enables the production of a coherent and robust assemblage 'addictive disorder' which incorporates psychological and social elements and exists beyond the specific consequences of drinking, smoking, using opiates and so on. Addictive disorder becomes an expansive category that can include rewarding non-drug activities such as gambling, eating and sex. However, this generalising approach exists in tension with another tradition of drug research, that of behavioural pharmacology, which focuses on the particular properties of different substances and their different levels of addictiveness and 'abuse potential' (Campbell 2007). This tension remains unresolved in generalised models of addiction because the substances they include are highly variable, not only in their effects and patterns of use, but in their legal and social status.

DSM: Diagnoses and disorders

The publication of the *DSM-III* in 1980 marked a paradigm shift in psychiatry from an era dominated by psychoanalytic theory to an official commitment to empiricism and scientific medicine. Unlike earlier psychiatric classification systems, the *DSM-III* established a diagnostic system based on specific and distinct categories of mental disorder (Wakefield 2006). These categories were based not on theories of causality but were produced from assemblages of observable and reportable symptoms. These clusters of symptoms were assumed to reflect discrete underlying disease conditions, but the manual itself was concerned with how these conditions appear rather than what causes them.

The focus on disease categories determined by appearances reflects one of the key aims of the developers of the *DSM-III*, which was to improve the reliability of psychiatric diagnosis. Reliability had been revealed to be embarrassingly deficient in several studies in the 1970s which found low levels of diagnostic agreement when the same patient was examined by different physicians (Kirk & Kutchins 1992). Concerns about diagnostic reliability are manifested in the technical rationality adopted in the manual. Each category has a code number and precise specifications about duration and inclusion and exclusion criteria. The numbered list of criteria for each condition constitutes psychiatric diagnosis as an objective rather than subjective exercise, with a clear-cut procedure to be applied by every professional in every case. However, as will become clear, subjective judgement remains an inevitable part of the evaluation of whether particular criteria are present or not.

Like all classificatory systems, the *DSM* constructs a certain reality through relations of similarity and difference (Jutel 2011). The approximately 400 conditions categorised in the *DSM-5* have in common their status as 'mental disorders', defined by a 'clinically significant disturbance in an individual's cognition, emotion, regulation, or behavior' which is associated with distress or disability (APA 2013a, 20). Thus, the manual enacts addiction as a condition more like depression or schizophrenia and less like other things, such as an everyday bad habit, a sin, a lifestyle or a physical disease such as an allergy. On the other hand, the manual places a boundary around addiction as a distinct disorder. Addiction may look like depression in some ways; it may cause depression or be caused by it, but it is distinct from depression because of its fundamental link with alcohol, drugs or intensely rewarding behaviours.

One of the biggest issues raised during the *DSM-5* revision process was the validity of the manual's categorical approach to illness, which defines discrete mental disorders with separate symptoms. Critics argued that clinical experience and biological research both suggested a much more dimensional reality, in which symptoms overlap and the borders between conditions such as depressive disorder and bipolar disorder or schizophrenia and obsessive-compulsive disorder (OCD) are blurred (Hyman 2007; First 2010; Adam 2013). These critics included eminent high-profile psychiatrists such as Steven Hyman, former head of the National Institute of Mental Health (NIMH). The high rates of co-morbidity found between different *DSM* conditions supported this view of a more fluid landscape of mental distress and dysfunction. The *DSM-5* acknowledges the limitations of the categorical approach in its introduction, stating that 'scientific evidence now places many... disorders on a spectrum with closely related disorders that have shared symptoms, shared genetic and environmental risk factors and possibly shared neural substrates...' (APA 2013a, 6). However, it retains the categorical approach, citing reasons of continuity, clarity and conciseness. Thus, the *DSM-5* is involved in a difficult ontological exercise: it is producing a reality (distinct mental diseases) which it admits is at odds with the reality of the world (a spectrum of overlapping dysfunctions).

Consistent with the categorical approach, the *DSM-5* presents mental disorders, such as the SUDs, in a tabular format with a numbered list of diagnostic criteria for each disorder. This results in a synchronic conceptualisation of addiction, in contrast to other enactments which present addiction as a process with a natural history that unfolds over time (most vividly seen in the Alcoholic Anonymous narrative of inexorable decline until rock bottom is reached) (Warhol & Michie 1996; Keane 2002). The textual effect of the *DSM* is of a snapshot, extracted from space and time, rather than a temporal process, although it is required that the symptoms be present for six months before a diagnosis is made.

Crucially, addiction is enacted in the *DSM* as an entity that is diagnosable: a checklist of symptoms is given, each of which a clinician can judge to be either present or absent in order to determine the relevance of the condition to the presenting individual. Unlike the *DSM-IV*, the *DSM-5* includes measurements of severity in an attempt to move towards a more dimensional conception of disorder. The presence of two or three symptoms indicates mild SUD, four or five symptoms moderate SUD and six or more severe SUD.

The process of diagnosis involves establishing medical authority over the condition and its treatment. It is not the subject who is able to judge the nature of the problem but the external and clinical gaze of the expert. Nevertheless, introspection and self-report is a crucial part of the diagnostic process. Some of the symptoms (such as withdrawal) may be exhibited by the patient, some (such as employment problems) may be a matter of record, but others are based on feelings, self-perception, intentions, forms of desire and aspects of cognition. For example, criterion 1 asks whether the substance is taken in larger amounts than intended, criterion 2 asks the patient whether there is a 'persistent desire' to cut down or control substance use and criterion 9 asks whether substance use is continued 'despite knowledge' of problems caused by the substance. As Room et al. (1996) have noted, such items assume a post-Enlightenment and reflective 'modern self' who stands outside of feelings and sensations and is able to evaluate and describe subjective states from an external viewpoint. Indeed, this self-aware and self-monitoring subject can be seen as one of the collateral realities produced by the diagnostic category.

What are clinicians identifying when they diagnose addiction using the *DSM*? In the next section we examine the 11 diagnostic criteria in turn. Before doing so, however, it is important to note that *DSM-5* installs a new core syndrome in the substance-related disorders chapter: 'substance use disorder'. This new syndrome replaces the two *DSM-IV* disorders of substance dependence and substance abuse and represents a significant change in addiction as a medical entity.

Substance use disorder is a rather ungainly entity composed of 11 heterogeneous criteria – all but one of the *DSM-IV* substance abuse items and all of the *DSM-IV* substance dependence items. The result is an increased diversity in symptoms of addiction and a proliferation of possible manifestations, given the disjunctive and polythetic nature of diagnosis in the *DSM* (polythetic refers to the fact that only some of the criteria need to be present in order for the diagnosis to be made). This has a potentially dramatic effect on how the disorder is enacted. It means that many subtypes of a single disorder are possible, with no single symptom necessarily shared by all who are diagnosed as 'dependent' (Room 1998, 313).

In an editorial explaining the advantages of the new category of SUD, Work Group member Marc Schuckit (2012) argued that the expanded criteria would address a wider range of patients, young and old, male and female, with different ethnic and class backgrounds. The generic nature of the disorder is also demonstrated by its ability to be converted into a list of ten distinct 'use disorders' such as opioid use disorder (shown in Table 1.2), tobacco use disorder, cannabis use disorder and so on. This heterogeneity produces a wide field of substance problems which moves addiction further away from the model of a discrete disorder based on a single underlying dysfunction. As noted earlier, the formula for a positive diagnosis now has a dimensional aspect. Diagnosis of a mild case requires only 2 of the 11 criteria. Such a low threshold has the potential to produce diagnostic bracket creep, resulting in a substantially increased prevalence of addictive disorders in the population. This is especially likely in the case of alcohol use, given the normative nature of frequent and high-volume drinking in particular groups such as students and young people (see Mewton et al. 2011).

The removal of substance abuse as a specific disorder was foreshadowed prior to the review by critics who argued that it contravened the requirement that mental disorders must not be merely examples of irresponsible or hazardous behaviour (Wakefield 2006; Martin et al. 2008). The disorder of substance abuse was supposed to capture cases of harmful drug use in the absence of dependence and therefore relied on 'symptoms' such as legal and personal problems. However, Charles O'Brien, head of the *DSM-5* Substance-Related Disorders Work Group, provided a different rationale for the elimination of the abuse category: a lack of data to support an intermediate state between drug use and drug addiction (O'Brien 2011, 866). Another rationale for the move from two disorders to one was that one set of criteria would be easier for clinicians to remember and use (Schuckit 2012). Items such as social and interpersonal problems and failure to fulfil role obligations have therefore not been removed from the diagnostic process with the deletion of substance abuse, rather they have been shifted into the new category of SUD.

The polythetic heterogeneity of the *DSM* model of addiction demonstrates its development from the alcohol dependence syndrome which was one of its most influential precursors (the alcohol dependence syndrome is discussed in more detail in Chapter 4). In the 1970s British psychiatrists Edwards and Gross (1976) put forward a 'provisional description' of the alcohol dependence syndrome which identified seven elements including withdrawal, tolerance and the subjective awareness of compulsion. In a later paper, Edwards (1986, 172) stated that the term 'syndrome' was used to imply 'the clustering of certain elements' and 'a co-occurrence with some coherence'. However, not all of the elements needed to be present for the syndrome to exist, and differences of degree between different elements could be expected. Thus despite Edwards and Gross's vision of some level of recognisable coherence in the construct of alcohol dependence, the syndromal concept contained in its structure the potential for disjunction and multiplicity. When operationalised in the *DSM*, the listing of independent elements enabled substance dependence to become broader in scope – to expand from the early focus in addiction medicine on alcohol and opiates to include substances such as cannabis, cocaine, nicotine, inhalants, hallucinogens and amphetamines. Such adaptability and expansiveness suit contemporary health management systems which require diagnosis for treatment: smokers, binge drinkers, patients who are dependent on prescription painkillers, heroin addicts and cannabis users can all be targeted for intervention. As we describe in Chapter 6, similar requirements contribute to changing understandings of overweight and obesity. But the classification of these substances as sharing a common addictive quality also shapes the way their use is conceptualised. There is a tendency to search for evidence of the substance dependence criteria in their patterns of use. For example, 'chain-smoking' is included as an example of the time-use criterion for tobacco use disorder, even though this form of continuous smoking often accompanies other forms of activity and is rarely a straightforward consumer of time (APA 2013a, 572).

Substance use disorder: The criteria

The *DSM-5* states that the 'essential feature' of SUD is 'a cluster of cognitive, behavioral, and physiological symptoms indicating that the individual continues using the substance despite significant *substance-related problems* [emphasis added]' (2013a, 483). As is the case in most medical models, this enactment of addiction places harm at the centre of the disorder. Specifically, a causal link must be established between drug use and various negative physical, psychological and social effects which are assembled into the entity 'substance-related problems'. As Mariana Valverde (1998) has observed, medical accounts of addiction demand a lot of work from the notion of harm, as it appears to promise an objective measure of dysfunction. Harm suggests that the problem is not the subjective and normative issue of excess (drinking or consuming more than is acceptable) but the consequences of the drinking or consuming and the subject's recognition of these consequences.

The *DSM-5* description then goes on to state that the diagnosis of an SUD is based on 'a pathological pattern of behaviors related to use of the substance' (2013a, 483). In the actual diagnostic categories for different substances this is called 'a problematic pattern' of use (see Table 1.2). This is a somewhat different notion from that of harm, as it suggests the existence of a pathology independent of observable negative consequences as well as the sense of a generally dysfunctional existence beyond the enumeration of specific symptoms. As is discussed below, not all the SUD diagnostic criteria are based on harm; the notion of risk and the idea of physiological disturbance are also incorporated into the disorder of addiction. Introducing a new level of organisation, the *DSM-5* divides the 11 criteria for SUD into four subgroups: *impaired control, social impairment, risky use* and *pharmacological criteria*. These are discussed in turn below.

Impaired control

Perhaps even more so than harmful use, loss of control or compulsion is a *sine qua non* of addiction. The addict is quintessentially a person whose choices and actions are no longer truly voluntary because addictive desire is both qualitatively and quantitatively distinct from normal desire. Indeed, it could be argued that harm has achieved its centrality in models of addiction because it is a way of identifying the compulsion that makes addiction a 'different state of being' from non-addiction (Leshner 2001). The addict's persistent repetition of self-damaging behaviour is interpreted as the sign of compromised autonomy, or to use older language, a diseased will (Valverde 1998). In the Alcoholics Anonymous understanding of addiction, the notion of the compromised will indicates a profound form of alienation in which the true self has been taken over by the disease of addiction (Denzin 1987; Keane 2000). The two SUD criteria which attempt to identify the existence of loss of control directly do not use the moralised and scientifically outmoded language of freedom of will or suggest such totalised alienation, but they identify a conflict within the self which bears the traces of this history.

Criterion 1 specifies that the substance be taken in larger amounts or over longer periods than intended, and criterion 2 that there is a persistent desire or unsuccessful efforts to cut down or control substance use. Both these criteria are reliant on self-report. In addition, criterion 1 demands clarity about the difference between what one hoped or planned to do and what happened, between decisions in the past and actions in the present. It also assumes that present perceptions of past intentions accurately reflect those past intentions. Underlying these assessments of failures of will is the culturally specific ideal of self-control and the belief that the individual exercise of self-discipline is the key to success and the achievement of a good life. As Robin Room has noted, addiction links loss of control over drinking or drug use with loss of control over the project of life in general:

> The concept is thus implicitly an explanation of perceived personal failure: the affected individual has failed to carry through on significant role expectations in his or her life; this failure is ascribed to a personal failure to control behaviour in accordance with expectations; and this loss of control is in turn ascribed to loss of control over drinking behaviour. (1985, 135)

Substance use disorder can be seen here to enact an important collateral reality: the proper, non-addicted individual as an autonomous agent who controls her level of consumption through conscious decisions. But drinking and drug use is a social practice structured by often powerful norms of reciprocity and sharing, as well as by the opportunistic seizing of experiences. Identifying 'taking in larger amounts than intended' as evidence of compulsion ignores documented social phenomena such as the 'controlled loss of control' sought in weekend drinking and which is incorporated into the project of life rather than derailing it (Measham & Brain 2005). Criterion 2 is similarly based on discordance between how subjects want to behave (to control or cut down use) and how they actually behave. This sense of a conflicted self, of contrary desires, of alienation from one's own behaviour, is a central feature of lay as well as medical understandings of addiction. By searching for conflict within the self and attributing it to a compulsive disorder, substance dependence produces another collateral reality: an ideal of health which depends on the existence of a unified and coherent internal self.

Criterion 3 is a less direct attempt to identify loss of control as it focuses on the individual's use or misuse of time. We will discuss it in the 'Social impairment' section below as it can be considered as much a matter of social impairment as of compulsion (although the *DSM* places it in the impaired control subgroup). Criterion 4 is that of craving or a 'strong desire' to use the substance. While this is the one new criterion that has been added to SUD from the existing *DSM-IV* dependence and abuse criteria, the concept of craving has a long history in addiction studies. Indeed, it is hard to imagine judging an individual as addicted without the presence of a strong desire for the substance (Kozlowski & Wilkinson 1987; Keane 2002). Along with terms such as compulsion and loss of control, the notion of craving signifies the strength of the forces directing the addict's behaviour, emphasising that addiction is outside normal experiences of desire, attachment and habit. Craving links this pathological intensity with a particular kind of problematic object, such as illicit drugs, implying that they produce an inherently different kind of desire. The inclusion of craving therefore represents continuity with earlier understandings of addiction.

Craving is frequently described in the scientific literature as a particularly difficult concept to define (Skinner & Aubin 2010). It is used both to describe an aversive state, part of the dysphoria of withdrawal, and a positive state, an anticipation of reward. It has been variously understood as produced by the absence of the drug, and its presence. However, with the ascendancy of the brain disease model of addiction, craving has been reconstituted as a neurobiological entity, identifiable as a particular pattern of brain activity visible via neuroimaging (World Health Organization 2004). Therefore its inclusion in the *DSM-5* criteria can be seen as over-determined; not just as continuity with earlier models, but as a response to brain-centred accounts of addiction. Neuropharmacological developments are particularly significant here. As Scott Vrecko (2010a) has argued, the development of 'brain-targeting' anti-craving medications such as naltrexone in the 1990s reinforced the idea that craving must be central to the process of addiction. Or to put this another way, if naltrexone is a solution to substance use and other compulsive behaviours, then these problems must be the result of craving-related brain abnormalities.

Social impairment

The *DSM-5* criteria grouped under social impairment are designed to capture the objective and observable harms produced by excessive substance use. But they reveal that the evaluation of harm is not a straightforward technical exercise, let alone the evaluation of use despite knowledge of harm. The criterion of occupational or educational harm caused by failure to fulfil 'major role obligations' (5) assumes certain middle-class norms of lifestyle, such as a structured routine of employment in which intoxication and/or absenteeism will result in economic loss and downward mobility (Valverde 1998). Criterion 6, which describes continued use despite social or interpersonal problems, assumes a social and intimate life which is external to drinking and drug use, rather than enmeshed with it.

Determining the extent to which the social impairment and associated harms experienced by drug-using individuals are 'substance-related problems' is not straightforward because of the variability of social context. For example, in highly marginalised populations such as the homeless injecting drug users studied by Bourgois and Schonberg (2009), harmful drug use is in one sense highly visible. However, Bourgois and Schonberg stress the structural nature of the extreme social and physical suffering experienced by these users, which is over-determined by poverty, unemployment, incarceration, dysfunctional social services and interpersonal violence as well as chronic alcohol and other drug use. Giving up alcohol and other drugs would not by itself ameliorate these conditions of existence; indeed, it could produce isolation from social networks. Moreover, many of the harms attributed to drugs are not caused directly by persistent drug use but by the legal status of specific drugs and the prohibitionist policies that have been enacted to control their use (Wodak 2007; Manderson 2011). By isolating individual patterns of substance use from particular social worlds and identifying them as the primary cause of suffering, the medicalised entity 'substance use disorder' enacts a reality in which individual acts and choices, and pre-determined effects of substances, produce misfortune and marginalisation, obscuring other realities of inequality and disadvantage.

In a different but related individualising impulse, two of the diagnostic criteria equate SUD with the mismanagement or misuse of time. These criteria rely on and reproduce culturally specific understandings of time as a commodity or resource and a socially specific context in which other more important and rewarding activities are in competition with substance use (Room 2003). Criterion 3 specifies that a 'great deal of time' is spent obtaining and using the substance or recovering from its effects. This requires a judgement about how much time is too much. For some, a weekly debilitating hangover could be a clear sign of excess and disorder; for others, an unremarkable feature of the weekend routine. The manual also states that in more severe cases 'virtually all of the individual's daily activities revolve around the substance' (APA 2013a, 483). Again, this statement assumes a clear separation between 'the substance' and daily activities, because the latter are seen to 'revolve around' the former. A different interpretation would not necessarily see socialising while drinking as a matter of social life revolving around alcohol, but rather life as an assemblage of multiple enmeshed practices taking place at one time.

Criterion 7 identifies harm in relation to the relinquishment of 'important social, occupational or recreational activities' because of substance use. The manual gives the example that 'the individual may withdraw from family activities and hobbies in order to use the substance' (APA 2013a, 483). Embedded in this example, and the criterion itself, is a hierarchical ranking of pleasures, in which family life and wholesome pursuits (assumed to be accessible and appealing to all) are placed above solitary consumption or the wrong sort of friends. Failure to order one's priorities in this way is designated a sign of disorder. This criterion is especially striking given the extensive literature on the intergenerational dimension to drug problems (Rhodes et al. 2003; Hayes et al. 2004).

Risky use

This group of criteria is interesting because – despite its designation – it combines a harm-based symptom, criterion 9, with a risk-based symptom, criterion 8. The common element is a focus on the physical consequences of substance use. Criterion 9, substance use despite knowledge of physical or psychological problems caused or exacerbated by the substance, raises difficulties similar to those associated with other harm-based symptoms. It is based on the identification of causality and awareness of that causality. While it is conceivable to argue that the physical and psychological problems experienced by marginalised drug users are exacerbated by their drug use, as we have already noted, the most powerful influences on their precarious existence could well lie elsewhere. Criterion 8, substance use in physically hazardous situations, comes from the *DSM-IV* substance abuse criteria, in which the example given is driving or operating machinery while affected by drugs. Here again we can see that an individual's vulnerability to addiction depends on social variables such as occupation (whether one's job requires the operation of machinery) and access to different forms of transport (for example, reliance on a car rather than public transport). It also raises questions about the status of other recreational activities which incur risk of physical harm without being pathologised, for example, horse-riding, fishing and mountain climbing (see Nutt 2009).

Pharmacological criteria

In medical models of addiction, a crucial element in the conversion of ideas of self-control and deficient will into a disease category is the identification of physiological dependence on the substance, as manifested by the existence of tolerance and withdrawal. In the *DSM-5*, tolerance and withdrawal (rebadged as pharmacological criteria rather than physical dependence) are the final two criteria (10 and 11). In the *DSM-IV* they were the first two criteria listed. Although all criteria are weighted equally irrespective of their place on this list, this positional decline from first to last is indicative of a significant downgrading in the role of dependence within scientific models of addiction. This shift is also seen in the abandonment of substance dependence as the name of addictive disorder, discussed in the following section.

The changed status of tolerance and withdrawal is especially noteworthy because until late last century physical dependence on a substance (such as alcohol or heroin) was regarded as the proof of genuine addiction. The delirium tremens of the alcoholic and sweating and cramps of the heroin addict were read as vivid signs of the physical otherness of the true addict. The scientists who established drug and alcohol studies in the mid-20th century relied heavily on physiological dependence to stabilise alcoholism and addiction as medical conditions and proper objects of scientific inquiry. For example, for E.M. Jellinek (1960), it was the presence of altered physiological responses, manifested in withdrawal and tolerance, which distinguished the disease of alcoholism from other forms of heavy drinking. Similarly, in 1957, the WHO committee on addiction-producing drugs emphasised physiological alteration as the basis of addiction when it set out two diagnostic categories, addiction and habituation, the former signifying the presence of both physical and psychological dependence, the latter 'only' psychological. This distinction demonstrated an enmeshment of the biological and the political, as it was in part an attempt to justify the subjection of some drugs (the addictive) but not others (the merely habit-forming) to strict international control (Room 1998, 310).

The privileging of physical dependence was reflected in the 1980 *DSM-III*, which required either tolerance or withdrawal for a diagnosis of substance dependence (Cottler et al. 1991). However, by the 1990s the growing influence of neuroscience made the physiological/psychological distinction seem a form of outmoded dualism. In 1993, the WHO Expert Committee on Drug Dependence stated that the distinction between physical and psychic dependence is 'not consistent with the modern view that all drug effects on the individual are potentially understandable in biological terms' (1993, 5). Since then neuroscientific knowledge of drug actions and reward mechanisms has further undermined distinctions between physical and psychological dependence by locating the brain as the source of all aspects of addiction, from withdrawal symptoms to the power of drug-linked places, people and things to provoke relapse in a former addict. The decreasing emphasis placed on physiological dependence as the pre-eminent indicator of addictive disease was also due to the result of increasing concern about drugs such as cocaine which did not have a clear-cut withdrawal syndrome.

In the *DSM-IV*, published in 1994, tolerance and withdrawal were neither necessary nor sufficient for a diagnosis of substance dependence and they had no more weight than the other criteria. Nevertheless, the distinction between the disorder of substance abuse (in which harmful drug use exists in the absence of dependence) and substance dependence continued to reinforce the salience of dependence as a marker of true addiction. Moreover, in the specifiers which followed the list of substance dependence criteria, a distinction was made between dependence with and dependence without physiological dependence. The condition with physiological dependence was described as 'associated with a more severe clinical course' for most classes of substances (APA 2000, 194). While the specifiers are gone in the *DSM-5*, the 2013 manual still notes that for most classes of substances, a history of withdrawal is associated with a 'more severe clinical course' (APA 2013a, 484).

In summary, the *DSM* model of addiction, now called SUD, produces addiction as a mental disorder in which a pattern of repeated and compulsive substance use produces significant physical, psychological and social harm. SUD assembles diverse elements such as harms, risk, misuse of time, loss of self-control, pathological desire and biological disturbance into the condition of addiction and locates it within the individual. However, as we have argued, the identification and evaluation of harm is not an objective or technical exercise as it involves judgements about what a meaningful and productive life looks like. In addition, harm does not exist in a vacuum but emerges from interactions between individual behaviour and the social. Like addiction or health or any other entity, harm can be seen as an assemblage of phenomena. From this point of view, distinguishing the object and its social context is less useful than recognising the particular forces and objects, including those less convenient or more costly to acknowledge, that must come together to produce harm. Another characteristic of the *DSM* model is that due to its disjunctive diagnostic formula (for example, meeting any four of the 11 criteria confirms a moderately severe disorder), it is theoretically possible that two people with the condition will not share a single symptom. Although it is presented as a single and unified entity, substance dependence can in fact be enacted in many different subtypes.

The end of dependence and the return of addiction

As noted previously, the *DSM-5* includes significant changes in the nomenclature of substance-related disorders. These changes are not just a matter of terminology but represent a redefining of addiction and a redrawing of its boundaries. The *DSM-5* reinstalls the language of addiction, which is not found in the *DSM-IV* (nor in the *DSM-III*), and removes substance dependence as the name of a disorder. Debates about 'addiction' versus 'dependence' as the designation for compulsive and harmful drug use were published during the *DSM-5* draft development process (Erickson & Wilcox 2006; O'Brien et al. 2006a, 2006b; Schuckit 2012). Supporters of the change to addiction in the *DSM-5* (including Charles O'Brien, the head of the Work Group) argued that 'substance dependence' was a confusing term which had promoted a lack of clarity about the difference between 'physical dependence' (that is, withdrawal and tolerance) and the disorder of compulsive and harmful drug use. While 'addiction' was seen by some as a stigmatising and unscientific term, O'Brien argued that its scientific acceptability was apparent in its widespread use in journal titles and the names of organisations such as the American Society of Addiction Medicine (O'Brien et al. 2006a).

The Work Group finally compromised by renaming the relevant chapter of the manual 'Substance-Related and Addictive Disorders' without using 'addiction' to designate an actual disorder. The manual explains that the word 'addiction' is not used as a diagnostic term because of its 'uncertain definition' and its 'potentially negative connotation'. The more 'neutral' term 'substance use disorder' is preferred because it can cover a wide range of disorder, from mild to severe. However, the manual notes that 'some clinicians will choose to use the word *addiction* [emphasis in original] to describe more extreme presentations' (APA 2013a, 485). By eschewing addiction as a diagnostic term, the *DSM-5* retains a distance from the neuroscientific discourse which routinely uses addiction to describe the brain disease of disrupted reward. As discussed previously, the generic term 'SUD' replaces substance dependence as the name of the condition of addictive drug use.

Despite the rather muted language, the naming of the chapter 'Substance-Related and Addictive Disorders' marks a major change in the constitution of addiction as a medical entity. It opens up the category of addiction to non-substance or behavioural addictions, an issue which has long been debated in the field (Orford 2001; Shaffer et al. 2004). In the *DSM-5*, the only behavioural addictive condition specifically included in the chapter is pathological gambling (renamed gambling disorder). In the *DSM-IV*, pathological gambling was classified as an impulse disorder and, although its diagnostic criteria remain largely the same, the shift into the addictive disorders category clearly represents a different understanding of the fundamental nature of the condition.

The only other behavioural addiction in the *DSM-5* is internet gaming disorder. It is not an officially recognised disorder, rather it appears in the chapter for 'conditions on which further research is encouraged' in order to inform decisions about inclusion in later editions of the manual (APA 2013a, 791). Obesity and compulsive sexuality were also proposed for inclusion as addictive conditions, but the relevant work groups decided that insufficient published data supported these changes (Volkow & O'Brien 2007; Kafka 2010; APA 2013b). However, the establishment of behavioural addictions in the manual makes theoretically possible a phalanx of new mental disorders based on failures of will and self-control, many related to everyday activities such as sex, exercise, shopping and eating.

The brain-based neurochemical model of addiction can be seen as one of the drivers of this expansionary approach to 'drug-independent addiction' (Vrecko 2010a, 40). Prevalent in the research on behavioural addictions is a neurobiological perspective in which a common neural dysfunction unites non-substance and substance addictions and in some sense renders the specific object of addiction irrelevant (see Shaffer et al. 2004; Potenza 2008). According to the APA, the rationale for grouping pathological gambling with drug addictions rests on the similarities in clinical expression, brain origin, comorbidity, physiology and treatment (2013b). The *DSM-5* itself states that 'gambling behaviors activate reward systems similar to those activated by drugs of abuse' (2013a, 481). Here we can see the radical potential of neuroscientific discourse in its ability to challenge the categories of licit and illicit and normal and pathological which have traditionally structured understandings of addiction.

While gambling disorder is grouped with substance disorders in the *DSM-5*, it is still constituted as different from these conditions because its object of addiction is not a drug. The substance use disorders are in a subsection titled 'Substance-Related Disorders' and are listed alphabetically from alcohol use disorder to tobacco use disorder, with the final entry being other (or unknown) substance use disorder. Gambling disorder follows in its own section, a section titled 'Non-Substance-Related Disorders', and while some of its diagnostic criteria related to loss of control are similar to those of the substance disorders, terms such as 'withdrawal' and 'tolerance' are not used. Furthermore, gambling disorder retains specific and unique criteria such as gambling while distressed, relying on others for money and 'chasing one's losses' which mark it out as different from alcohol and other drug addictions.

The point here is that while the brain disease model focuses on the disrupted reward system which it views as underlying all addictions, the *DSM-5* retains an object-focused approach in which each addictive object (alcohol, opiates, tobacco, gambling and so on) has its own designated disorder. Moreover, it divides these disorders according to a drug/non-drug binary and therefore reinforces the existence of 'drugs' as a particularly problematic and powerful category of things (see Chapter 6 for more on the enactment of the category of 'drugs' in the neuroscience of obesity). In this way, the radical potential of neuroscientific discourse to challenge categories of normal and pathological forms of desire and consumption is forestalled.

Another rationale given for the shift from dependence to addiction in the *DSM-5* also demonstrates a continuing commitment to constituting drug addicts and drug addiction as different from other forms of disordered consumption. In the lead-up to the *DSM-5*, O'Brien argued that the decision to adopt 'substance dependence' in the *DSM-III* was a serious mistake because it promoted confusion between the disorder of compulsive and uncontrolled drug use and the physiological condition of dependence which is 'a normal physiological adaptation to repeated dosing of a medication' (O'Brien et al. 2006a, 764). According to O'Brien (2011, 867), the most deleterious effects of this bad decision have been suffered by pain patients who have been stigmatised and denied adequate treatment because dependence on opiates has been wrongly equated with addiction. Thus in the *DSM-5*, the criteria of tolerance and withdrawal are explicitly not to be counted towards diagnosis of SUD if they occur in those taking medications such as opiates, sedatives and stimulants under medical supervision (see Table 1.2) (APA 2013a, 484).

As a result of this exclusion, one of the collateral realities enacted by the latest *DSM* revision is a reinforced distinction between medically produced drug dependence and illicit and recreationally produced drug dependence. The symptoms of dependence, withdrawal and tolerance, which used to be the markers of genuine addiction, have become polysemic signifiers whose meaning is dependent on the absence or presence of medical supervision. Medical authority renders them expected side-effects of treatment, while outside the clinical space, when combined with certain social realities, they become signs of compulsive and disordered desire. The normalisation of physiological dependence when it occurs as a result of medically authorised opiate use has important effects on the substance of drugs themselves. In the *DSM-5*, the pharmacological similarities between prescription medications and drugs such as heroin are rendered less salient than the different contexts of their use. A complicating factor here is the increasing prominence of 'prescription painkiller abuse' as an illicit drug problem and public health threat, a phenomenon which destabilises the boundary between medications and illicit recreational drugs (Compton & Volkow 2006; Quintero 2012).

This is not just a matter of symptoms and their interpretation. The insistence that medically authorised opiate users should be excluded from the stigmatised category of addiction produces addicts as individuals who deserve stigmatisation and belong in this devalued category.[3] Therefore, while one effect of the *DSM* is to medicalise addiction as 'substance use disorder', it also acts to reinforce moralised categories of legitimate and illegitimate drug use.

DSM-5 debates

One of the collateral effects of the *DSM-5* process was a flourishing of critical commentary which not only addressed the validity of particular disorders but took aim at the descriptive approach to nosology and diagnosis operationalised in the *DSM*. The descriptive approach, first adopted in the *DSM-III*, was originally celebrated for its eschewal of speculative causal explanations in favour of clusters of observable symptoms; at the time, this shift was seen as a move to a more reliable and scientific paradigm (Kirk & Kutchins 1992; First 2010). However, as the *DSM-IV* approached the end of its active life, and the capacity of neuroscience to identify and explain psychopathological processes was seen to be increasing, the limitations of descriptive nosology and its failure to 'carve nature at its joints' became increasingly frequent topics in psychiatric literature. Steven Hyman (2010, 169 and 171) listed fundamental problems with the current system, including 'arbitrary and rigid' thresholds, excessive co-morbidity and inconsistencies with the data emerging from genetic and family studies.

Given these frustrations and the sense that psychiatry was losing scientific credibility, it is not surprising that a primary aim of the *DSM-5* revision was to move towards a pathophysiological classificatory system based on neurobiology, brain imaging and genetics (Charney et al. 2002; Kupfer et al. 2002). The research agenda published in phase one of the process stated that the ultimate goal was a system based on the translation of neuroscience research into nosology which was likely to be 'radically different' from the current approach (Charney et al. 2002, 70). However, despite the scientific optimism of some of the early commentary and the glowing coverage of advances in biomedical research, a few years later most experts seem to have concluded that it was too early to include information about brain structure and function into the *DSM* (Hyman 2007).

The *DSM-5* reflects this tension between the desire for a new neuroscientific nosology and the awareness of the limits of the existing research data. It contains general statements about the lack of 'fully validated diagnoses' in previous versions of the manual and the 'real and durable' progress made in neuroscience, brain imaging, genetics and epidemiology since the *DSM-IV* (APA 2013a, 5). However, it adds that the science of mental disorders is continuing to evolve and 'speculative results do not belong in an official nosology' (5).[4]

Certainly, as in the case of the substance-related disorders, *DSM-5* diagnosis remains based on the subjective evaluation of behaviour and reported experiences and feelings, despite the increasing authority of the brain disease model of addiction. But in contrast to the behavioural and social measures of harmful drug use found in the diagnostic criteria, the first paragraph of the 'Substance-Related and Addictive Disorders' chapter constitutes SUD as fundamentally a dysfunction of the brain. It states that addiction occurs because drugs of abuse produce such an 'intense activation of the reward system' that normal activities are neglected (APA 2013a, 481). Later, the relapsing nature of SUD is attributed to 'an underlying change in brain circuits that may persist beyond detoxification' (483).

Despite these enactments of neural substrates, the lack of a move to more precise biological criteria in the *DSM-5* has produced a collateral reality of uncertainty which contrasts with the rhetoric of scientific progress towards unity and clarity. Marc Schuckit (2012, 521), a member of the APA Substance-Related Disorders Work Group, explained in an editorial that biological tests would not be included because 'the truth of the matter is that, similar to many medical and psychiatric conditions, the essence of the SUDs has not yet been clearly identified'. He described current understanding of these disorders as a 'blurry image' and cited the parable of the blind men and the elephant (a familiar epistemological trope, as we will see in Chapter 5, in debates about alcohol addiction), suggesting that it was important not to discard earlier research just to move to another perspective.

Before the *DSM-5* was even published, it attracted devastating and widely publicised criticisms focused on its conceptualisation of mental disorders. In what was described as a 'bombshell' of 'potentially seismic proportions', the US government's NIMH, the world's largest mental health research organisation, distanced itself from the *DSM* (Underwood 2013). NIMH director Thomas Insel denounced the manual's lack of scientific validity and its continued reliance on outdated symptom-based diagnosis (Insel 2013). Stating that patients with mental disorders 'deserve better', he announced that the NIMH would be 're-orienting its research away from DSM categories' in order to focus on the production of objective data based on genetics, imaging and cognitive science. To replace the *DSM* it would develop its own biologically valid framework for research, diagnosis and treatment, the Research Domain Criteria project. This new classification system would begin from the assumption that 'mental disorders are biological disorders involving brain circuits' (Insel 2013).

Taking the opposite position, the British Psychological Society (BPS) used the publication of the *DSM-5* to challenge the biomedical model of mental illness as disease and to argue for a more interdisciplinary and contextualised understanding of psychological distress (Division of Clinical Psychology 2013). The society's division of clinical psychology issued a consensus statement in May 2013 stating that disease-based psychiatric classification systems, such as the *DSM*, had significant theoretical, empirical and ethical flaws which undermined evidence-based practice and research. The statement calls for a recognition of 'the complex range of life experiences' and 'social and relational circumstances' that produce mental distress (Division of Clinical Psychology 2013). In many ways this statement can be read as a continuation of a long-standing conflict between humanistic psychology and biological psychiatry, in this case also informed by the different traditions of UK and US mental health treatment. The publication of the *DSM-5*, with its unfulfilled neurobiological aspirations, has, it seems, forced these divisions within the psy disciplines to the fore.

These criticisms of the *DSM-5* highlight the fact that mental disorders are assembled and disassembled from social, political and technical processes that determine what is to count as scientific fact in particular times and locations. While both the NIMH and the BPS argue that the *DSM* has failed to capture the reality of mental illness, the processes involved in producing the *DSM-5* were as much about negotiation and consensus building between experts as about scientific validation (Edwards 2012; Schuckit 2012). In the final two sections of this chapter we focus specifically on the model of addiction as a brain disease, highlighting the processes involved in stabilising another authoritative version of disordered desire and consumption.

Addiction neuroscience: A closer look

As we have indicated, the medicalisation, or indeed biomedicalisation, of addiction moved into a new stage with the development of the brain disease model in the late 20th century. As Nancy Campbell (2012, 19) has argued, the US National Institute on Drug Abuse (NIDA) recast addiction as 'an exemplary proving ground' on which to demonstrate the translational value of neuroscience, thereby refiguring addiction as a primarily molecular process. However, as discussed in this section, neurochemical explanations of addiction remain limited and partial. In particular, the question of how molecular processes translate into complex social behaviours and practices remains open (Campbell 2012).

The model of addiction as a 'chronic relapsing brain disease' emerged out of a confluence of scientific, technical and political developments, most particularly an alliance between addiction science and US drug control in the mid-20th century. When drug use was politically targeted as a key element of social disorder and crisis in the 1970s, one government response was the funding of basic addiction research that enabled researchers to bring into being new biological truths about drug receptors and neurotransmitters (Courtwright 2010; Vrecko 2010b). At the same time, the development of imaging technologies enabled the brain to be studied more easily and cheaply, without the need for post-mortem human tissue (Campbell 2007). As Vrecko (2010b, 61) writes, researchers were able to form a new 'neurobiological problem space' and situate addiction within it. Facts about receptors, drugs and brain dysfunction were brought into being and entered into 'practical and political trajectories' connected with drug control, abstinence-based treatments and anti-drug education (see also Elam 2012).

By locating addiction within the brain and identifying it as a brain disease, neuroscience produces it as a fundamentally biological process. Visual representations have been central to the localisation of addiction in the inner neurological space of the individual (Keane 1999; Dumit 2004). Positron emission tomography (PET) scans, which show addiction as a particular pattern of colour contrasted with the different pattern which denotes the 'healthy brain', have become a feature not only of research articles but of educational material and public health campaigns warning of the dangers of drug use. But these vivid images of localisation are combined with an expansionary understanding of the biological which enables 'brain processes' to incorporate all relevant aspects of psychological and social experience, from memory, mood and affect to intention, risk-taking and self-perception. In the brain disease model, social and cultural features are acknowledged, often in phrases such as 'addiction is not *just* [emphasis added] a brain disease' (Leshner 1997, 46). But, as we will see in later chapters, they are either relegated to the vague background realm of 'environmental influences' or refigured as effects of disordered brain chemistry. For example, the propensity of teenagers to experiment with drugs and their vulnerability to addiction is explained as a consequence of incomplete development of brain regions and different forms of neuroadaptation (Volkow & Li 2004).

One collateral reality enacted here is the stabilisation of 'the brain' as complex and plastic enough to explain variable human experiences such as addiction, but also straightforward and fixed enough to be reduced to simple explanatory models. In addition, the plasticity of the brain is presented as rendering it open to change in both function and structure in response to stimulation, such as the powerful stimulation of drugs. However, the brain disease model also produces a certain rigidity as characteristic of the addicted brain. The changes produced by long-term drug use are frequently described as remarkably enduring if not permanent, persisting well beyond the period of active drug use (Hyman & Malenka 2001; Leshner 2001; American Society of Addiction Medicine 2013).

The central player in this enactment of addiction is 'the brain reward system' which is damaged by long-term drug consumption. The explanatory narrative that has been distilled and stabilised from the complex neuroscience of drugs and reward is a simple one, strengthened by the appeal of evolutionary logic. The story is that the brain's reward system evolved in order to reinforce 'survival-relevant natural goals' such as searching for food, eating and sex (Hyman 2005).

Specifically, these activities produce pleasure via the release of the neurotransmitter dopamine which binds 'the hedonic properties of a goal to desire and to action' (Hyman 2005, 1416). Addictive drugs are able to 'hijack' this reward system because while they act in a similar way to natural rewards, they produce an artificially intense and rapid positive response (Robinson & Berridge 2003). The brain adapts to the presence of a drug by remodelling synapses and circuits, further increasing the reinforcing effects of the drug. Because of these long-lasting neural changes the addict is regarded as existing in 'a different state of being', in which drugs are the highest motivational priority and other goals and relationships are abandoned (Leshner 2001, 76).

As is explored in more detail later in relation to different substances, an important collateral reality stabilised in this account of the 'hijacked brain' is a unified category of drugs as the things which instantiate the process of addiction. Steven Hyman's (2005, 1415) explanation demonstrates a typical move from diversity to singularity: 'Addictive drugs represent diverse chemical families, stimulate or block different initial molecular targets, and have many unrelated actions outside the ventral tegmental area/nucleus accumbens circuit, but through different mechanisms they all ultimately increase synaptic dopamine within the nucleus accumbens.'

The neuroscientific discourse of addiction is replete with seemingly interchangeable phrases such as 'addictive drugs', 'all drugs of abuse', 'all psychoactive substances' to describe the substances that produce the relevant effects in the brain (often referred to as 'drug-induced brain changes'). In turn these changes result in 'drug-craving' and 'drug-seeking'. But the category of drugs is taken for granted and not explicitly defined; are all psychoactive substances addictive? Is 'drugs of abuse' a socio-legal or natural-chemical category? It seems both types of category are being assembled into addiction here. In order to produce particular brain responses, the relevant substances must share some common chemical properties, but the 'aberrant behaviours' of drug-seeking and 'drug-craving' are identified with particular socially demonised and illicit substances. This stabilisation and privileging of the category 'drugs' occurs at the same time as a seemingly contrary expansion of potential addiction triggers to include non-drug rewards such as food, gambling and sex. This tension is managed through the refiguring of non-drug rewards as drug-like in their effects. As outlined in Chapter 6, for example, the neuroscientific literature on obesity frequently categorises sugar, refined carbohydrates, fat and salt as 'addictive substances'.

Another important characteristic of the brain disease model is a focus on positive appetitive reward as the driver of the addictive process. This contrasts with earlier pre-molecular understandings that identified withdrawal as the marker of genuine, physiological dependence. In this earlier model of addiction as disease, the addict sought drugs primarily to avoid or alleviate the aversive effects of withdrawal (Jellinek 1960; Solomon 1977). Thus while drug use may have originally been pleasurable, the development of dependence shifts the process to one of negative reinforcement. However, while neuroscience places reward at the core of addiction, this is not a simple notion of the experience of pleasure or euphoria. Rather, current neuroscientific discourse tends to separate liking from wanting, positing that dopamine release maintains the state of 'wanting' a drug that may be independent from 'liking' its effects (Hyman 2005; Berridge 2007; Pelchat 2009). Thus, similar to the 'withdrawal avoidance' model, drug addicts are enacted as disordered individuals driven to continue a practice they no longer enjoy.

Neurochemical normality and disorder

In contrast to the *DSM,* which enacts addiction as a mental disorder located in the same classificatory system as entities such as mood and personality disorders, the brain disease model stabilises a different set of relationships. In their account of addiction as 'the neurobiology of behavior gone awry', NIDA scientists Volkow and Li invoke an organic vision of the disease:

> [D]rug addiction is a disease of the brain, and the associated abnormal behaviour is the result of dysfunction of brain tissue, just as cardiac insufficiency is a disease of the heart and abnormal blood circulation is the result of dysfunction of myocardial tissue. (2004, 963)

This brain/heart analogy is supported by an illustration which symmetrically juxtaposes PET scans of a healthy brain and an addicted brain and PET scans of a healthy heart and a heart damaged by myocardial infarction. The caption instructs readers to

> note the decreased glucose metabolism in the OFC (orbitofrontal cortex) of the addicted person and the decreased metabolism in the myocardial tissue in the person with a myocardial infarct. Damage to the OFC will result in improper inhibitory control and compulsive

> behaviour, and damage to the myocardium will result in improper blood circulation. (2004, 964)

The echoing of terms and phrases (decreased metabolism, damage to the X will result in improper Y) produces addiction as a physiological rather than psychological phenomenon, as incontrovertible, concrete and physically present in the body as heart disease.

Nevertheless, Volkow and Li shift from terms like 'improper inhibitory control' to 'aberrant behaviour', producing brain disease as a biological reality that can be readily assembled with the behavioural and social criteria of the *DSM* in a cause-and-effect relationship. In this way the brain is not like the heart; it can be read as equivalent to the self – a disordered brain equals a disordered self and a disordered life. The identification of an underlying neural dysfunction that causes the many different manifestations of substance use disorder, from the craving for a cigarette to the symptoms of heroin withdrawal, has a powerful unifying effect. Underneath the heterogeneity of SUD, with its 11 criteria and its multitude of subtypes, is a singular truth of addiction. But there is a circularity and interiority in this relationship which is masked by the attribution of cause and effect. The brain disease model begins with the problem of addiction as defined by the medical discourse of harm and compulsion and seeks to explain it. For example, the idea that synapses are remodelled so that drugs take on 'the highest motivational priority' and other goals are abandoned can be seen as a biologised re-telling of the *DSM* social and occupational harm criterion. Moreover, the narrative of the 'hijacked brain' with its division of activities into the natural and authentically rewarding (eating, heterosexual sex and socialising) and the artificially and preternaturally pleasurable (drugs) relies on the same normative ordering represented in the *DSM* criteria, in which disorder is manifested by a loss of interest in family and a devotion to solitary substance use. Thus, despite their professed moral neutrality, neurochemical explanations of addiction continue to reflect and reproduce the pathological figure of the addict whose life has been destroyed by the inherently destructive power of drugs. And rather than being prior to the hybrid *DSM* assemblage, the brain disease model is reliant on it for its conceptual content and salience.

Unlike the *DSM* model, the neuroscientific account of addiction stresses an anatomical and binary difference between the addict and the non-addict (as in the Volkow and Li illustration). This is a powerful 'neuroscience of difference' in which the addict's deviance from the norm goes much deeper than surface aberrations of behaviour, and lasts much longer than the duration of the observable signs of disorder (Buchman et al. 2010). Chronicity and durability are emphasised in the brain disease model: an altered brain leaves the addict prone to relapse long after drug use has ceased. The assertion that an addict is a different kind of human being, and has become so as a result of choices about consumption, is at odds with the belief that the brain disease model will undermine the stigma of addiction (Buchman et al. 2010). It produces addicts' 'aberrant behaviour' as evidence of otherness rather than of responses to the particular circumstances and predicaments of their lives.

However, there is an instability in this enactment of addiction. The molecular style of thought found in the brain disease model has the potential to destabilise as well as reinforce the difference of the addict. Because it is the 'natural' affinity between drugs and the brain that explains why people take psychoactive substances and why some find it impossible to stop, the narrative of the hijacked brain can be interpreted as a normalising account of addiction. It suggests that normal brains have an inherent capacity for addiction, challenging earlier theories of addiction as a kind of personality disorder or character flaw. For example, in its lengthy report on the neuroscience of substance use and dependence, the World Health Organization (WHO) describes the action of substances in the brain as part of 'the common biological inheritance shared by all humans' and states that substance dependence is 'a medical disorder that could affect any human being' rather than a sign of weakness (2004, 242, 248). Nikolas Rose (2003, 2007) has emphasised the normalising potential of neurochemical explanations of addiction, arguing that they construct the problem as a correctible error rather than a deep, resistant and pervasive pathology. In his view, neurochemistry renders addiction an anomaly rather than an abnormality and thereby promises to lift the moral weight that characterises earlier disease models.

The neuroscientific account's emphasis on the common neural effects of psychoactive substances does bring into question the socio-legal categorisation of psychoactive substances into medications, illicit drugs and legal substances. As the WHO report points out, from a neuroscientific perspective it is unclear why heroin, cocaine, cannabis and amphetamines are subject to international conventions which outlaw their use, while alcohol is not (2004, 37). Similarly, to return to the *DSM-5*, the distinction between the opiate dependence of the pain patient and the opiate dependence of the addict is not supported by any reference to neurological difference. Moreover, the brain disease model suggests that the pleasure drugs produce is not qualitatively different from that generated by rewards such as food, sex and social interaction, because these experiences are all mediated through dopamine. Drugs are harmful precisely because the effects they induce are enough like healthy pleasures to act as substitutes for them. The recognition of behavioural addictions in the *DSM-5* is consistent with this assemblage of drug and non-drug rewards as it acknowledges the possibility of drug-independent compulsions which are as powerful and potentially harmful as drug dependence. In this expanded form, addiction can be re-imagined as a problem of the majority rather than confined to a marginalised minority. It is a problem that can develop from activities that are not only morally neutral but positively valued and encouraged (such as exercise, healthy eating and work). As suggested in Chapters 6 and 7, the increasing emphasis on food as a psychoactive substance raises further questions about existing distinctions between drugs and opens new debates about the trajectory of addiction as aberrant or pathological.

But despite its bringing together of drug and 'natural' rewards, the disruptive potential of the brain disease model is constrained by the other entrenched medical, social and legal assemblages that constitute and regulate drugs and drug use. As historian David Courtwright (2010) points out, the brain model has achieved cultural prominence as a scientific theory, but its clinical influence has so far been limited, and neither has it challenged the dominance of prohibitionist drug policy in the United States. In Alan Leshner's (2001) widely cited article, 'Addiction is a Brain Disease', we can see how readily neuroscience is incorporated into pre-existing visions of the addict as a profoundly disordered individual. While Leshner (2001, 80), then head of the NIDA, argues for the importance of treatment and a public health approach in this article, he simultaneously supports existing systems of drug control in order to stem the supply of drugs that he describes as the agents of disease. In the WHO neuroscience report, a similar kind of tension exists between the constitution of addiction as a chronic medical disorder that could affect anyone and the framework of the United Nations drug conventions which is described but not explicitly challenged.

The WHO report ends with a chapter on ethical issues raised by the neuroscience of addiction, and the conclusion includes the statement that 'regardless of the level of substance use and which substance an individual takes, they have the same rights to health, education, work opportunities and reintegration into society, as does any other individual' (2004, 248). The notion of 'reintegration into society', converted here into a right rather than a duty, assumes that society is a single entity and that drug users are external to it. But despite the invocation of a human rights framework, the discussion of ethics is dominated by traditional bioethical issues such as informed consent, participation in research, access to genetic information and coerced treatment. Apart from noting in one sentence that arguments against drug criminalisation are couched in ethical terms, the report excludes the discussion of drug control from its ontology of the ethical. The human rights of substance users briefly invoked in the conclusion thereby remain a transient and undeveloped element in the reality of addiction.

Conclusion

In this chapter we have outlined the stabilisation of addiction as a disease in contemporary medicine. We focused on two influential phenomena, the addictive disorder categorised in the new edition of the APA's diagnostic manual and the chronic, relapsing, brain disease model currently dominating addiction science. Both versions reveal the way that addiction operates to shape the varied problems and predicaments of alcohol and other drug use (and broader social ills) into an entity located within the individual. The addicted individual is thus realised as a target for particular forms of regulation and intervention in order to restore the idealised state of autonomy, control and productivity reified as normal and healthy existence.

The now-superseded *DSM-IV* model of substance dependence reflected a clinical tradition of conceptualising addiction in relation to harm and diagnosing it through the presence of a collection of observable and reportable symptoms. The emphasis on repeated drug use producing harm as the indicator of pathology, rather than repeated drug use per se, was supposed to guarantee the objectivity of the diagnostic process. However, this evaluation of harm necessarily involves a subjective assessment of how far a life has deviated from a norm of healthy and prudent living. The symptoms of dependence associated with compulsion and the misuse of time also enact an ideal of autonomous agency in which levels and patterns of consumption are controlled by the individual and are subordinate to more socially valued priorities.

While the *DSM-5* contains a significant revision of substance-related disorders as presented in the *DSM-IV*, the diagnosis remains based on the subjective evaluation of behaviour and reported experiences and feelings. It proposes a new core syndrome 'substance use disorder' which merges the *DSM-IV* disorders of substance dependence and substance abuse. Because SUD has 11 criteria (not all of which must be met for a positive diagnosis), it represents an increased diversity of symptoms of addiction and a proliferation of possible manifestations. This heterogeneity produces a wide field of substance problems, moving addiction further away from the model of a discrete disorder based on a single underlying dysfunction.

The removal of the term 'dependence' as the name of a disorder and the re-installation of the language of addiction in the *DSM-5* represents an important shift in the remaking of addiction. The use of the title 'Substance Use and Addictive Disorders' for the relevant section of the manual opens the category of addiction to non-substance compulsions. This recognition of 'drug-independent' addictions has in part been driven by the neuroscientific research that has dominated addiction science for the past two decades. By refiguring addiction as dysfunction of the brain's reward system, the brain disease model of addiction has challenged the distinction between pleasure derived from 'natural' rewards such as food and sex and the pleasures of drugs. While the latter are still understood as artificially intense and therefore able to 'hijack' the brain, the former are also potentially addictive because they produce similar dopaminergic effects.

Advocates of the brain disease model argue not only for its scientific validity but for its ethical effects. According to Nora Volkow, the head of NIDA, recognition of the neurobiology of addiction will undermine the stigmatisation of addicts and replace punishment with treatment (Volkow & Li 2004). However, medicalisation does not necessarily lead to de-stigmatisation, and powerful social and legal forces continue to invest addiction with moral weight. Drug use, especially illicit drug use, continues to be understood as an inherently suspect form of consumption. The reductionism of the brain disease model enables it to produce elegant and productive facts about molecular effects, but it is ill-equipped to make meaningful connections between the interior space of the brain, the lived experience of addiction and socio-material networks of consumption and health. As we show in later chapters, both the *DSM* and the neuroscience of addiction remake addiction in new and familiar ways, enacting numerous important collateral realities – 'drugs' as a cohesive category, the subject of health as unified and self-aware, the body as stable, the social 'context' or 'environment' as a simple set of variables or influences – along the way.

2
Stabilising Stimulants: Amphetamine Dependence and Methamphetamine Addiction

Alcohol and heroin have traditionally been constituted as the classic drugs of addiction. In recent years, however, the amphetamines, a group of synthetic stimulant drugs, have assumed an increasingly prominent place in debates on addiction. In this chapter, we explore influential psychological and neuroscientific research on amphetamine and methamphetamine as case studies in changing realities of addiction. We argue, in turn, that 'amphetamine dependence' in the 1990s and 'methamphetamine addiction' in the 2000s emerged in repeated and vigorous research attempts to define them as stable objects for policy and practice purposes. In tracing this process of definition and stabilisation, we identify a range of crucial changes in the meanings of, and collateral realities enacted in, addiction, with the most significant being that the definition of addiction was revised to emphasise its psychological component and to encompass a wider range of drug use patterns. We also consider the collateral realities constituted in the neuroscience of methamphetamine, which has increasingly come to be invoked as an explanatory paradigm, in order to highlight its emerging role in research attempts to stabilise and extend the application of methamphetamine addiction to various patterns of consumption.

Tracing these processes of stabilisation, extension and explanation, and identifying their political effects, is important because they have the potential to dramatically reshape understandings of the social and health issues relating to amphetamine and methamphetamine, allowed increasing numbers of drug consumers to be pathologised and powerfully remade ideas about addiction. However, as we show in the next chapter, they have so far led to few specific changes in policy and treatment. In later chapters, we contrast the vigour and success of psychological and neuroscientific research attempts to define and stabilise amphetamine dependence and methamphetamine addiction with the volatility, ambiguity and instability of definitions of alcohol addiction, and the recent emergence of neuroscientific attempts to enact obesity as yet another form of addiction. We begin this chapter by tracing the background to recent growth in concern about amphetamine and methamphetamine and reviewing previous sociological work on these drugs.

Concern about methamphetamine

Methamphetamine is sometimes described as a more powerful, purer version of amphetamine; at other times it is conflated with amphetamine. International concern in research, policy and public discourse about the scale and effects of amphetamine use peaked in the 1990s, while concern about methamphetamine peaked in the 2000s. Whether the particular concerns expressed were warranted remains a contested issue. Klee noted:

> The 1990s decade started with news of major developments worldwide in amphetamine use that are likely not only to have implications for the regions affected but also for the nature and style of illicit drug markets in the future. (2001, 22)

Klee explains that 1995 saw the start of a series of international meetings aimed at assessing the scale and possible effects of these developments. In 1996, for example, the United Nations Drug Control Programme (UNDCP) met in Vienna, finding that amphetamine use was indeed growing in scale and intensity. It reported that amphetamines were the second most popular illegal substances in the world after cannabis, and predicted further expansion in use. Production and trafficking were reported to be exceeding all measures of control.

Since the 1990s, epidemiological research has reported increases in the use of amphetamine and methamphetamine and related health and social problems in many parts of the world (for example, North America, South East Asia and Australia). This research, particularly that focused on methamphetamine, has been accompanied by extensive media coverage, legislative change, parliamentary inquiries, international meetings, and the development of specific policy and practical responses. In the process, many strong claims have been made about the characteristics and extent of methamphetamine (as opposed to amphetamine) use, with a particular focus on crystalline methamphetamine or 'ice' (headlines favour puns and hyperbole: 'ice storm', 'ice age', a 'bigger threat than terrorism'). These claims have focused on the attributes and capacities of those who use the drug (they are 'crazed', 'dangerous', 'psychotic', 'devastated', 'destroyed'), on the properties of the drug itself (more 'addictive' than heroin, 'potent', 'pure', 'ultra-powerful') and on the scale and nature of the health and social problems – such as addiction and dependence – deemed to be associated with its use ('epidemic', 'battleground', 'overwhelming' emergency services).

Public discourse on methamphetamine use articulates in many different settings and modes a sense of crisis, drama and emergency, as can be seen in three examples taken from respected news media sources. The first example refers to the wave of concern about methamphetamine's potential impact in Hawaii in 1989. In the words of the Chief of the Honolulu Police Department, as reported in the broadsheet *Weekend Australian* newspaper: 'The Ice problem is so bad that Crack [an infamous cocaine derivative] pales by comparison. Ice is cheaper to produce, and is more addictive than heroin' (Safe & Sager 1990, 11). The second and third examples come from a later moment of intense concern – the mid-2000s. The first is an extract from an Australian Broadcasting Corporation web page promoting an Australian television documentary entitled 'The Ice Age', aired on 20 March 2006:

> It's cheap, highly addictive and ultra-powerful. 'Ice', or crystal methamphetamine, is now more popular than heroin, playing havoc with the minds and bodies of nearly 50,000 Australians. Ice is filling emergency wards with psychotic, dangerous patients, to the alarm of doctors who thought they'd seen everything. 'They're the most out of control, violent human beings I have ever seen in my life – and I've been around for a long time', says one. 'It makes heroin seem like the really good old days'.
>
> (Accessed on 2 August 2013: www.abc.net.au/4corners/content/2006/s1593168.htm)

The third example is provided by US Attorney General Alberto Gonzales, who, in 2005, said that 'in terms of damage to children and to our society, meth[amphetamine] is now the most dangerous drug in America' (*Newsweek*, 8 August 2005). The Gonzales quotation appears in a *Newsweek* article that carries the following sub-heading:

> **[METH] CREATES A POTENT, LONG-LASTING HIGH – UNTIL THE USER CRASHES AND, TOO OFTEN, LITERALLY BURNS.**

HOW METH QUIETLY MARCHED ACROSS THE COUNTRY AND UP THE SOCIOECONOMIC LADDER – AND THE WRECKAGE IT LEAVES IN ITS WAKE. AS LAW ENFORCEMENT FIGHTS A LOSING BATTLE ON THE GROUND, OFFICIALS ASK: ARE THE FEDS DOING ALL THEY CAN TO CONTAIN THIS EPIDEMIC?

(Accessed on 2 August 2013: www.thedailybeast.com/newsweek/2005/08/08/america-s-most-dangerous-drug.html, original capitalisation and bolding)

The emergence in the 1990s and 2000s of this heightened language regarding methamphetamine use has been criticised by several scholars as constituting a 'moral panic'. In 1993, Lauderback and Waldorf (1993), for example, examined the warnings against the dangers of crystalline methamphetamine issued by various government agencies in the late 1980s on the basis of its reputed popularity in Hawaii. These dangers included methamphetamine's potency, addiction potential and risk of paranoid schizophrenia. They compared these 'portents of doom' with available research evidence in California, the nearest mainland US state to Hawaii, and found that the use of crystalline methamphetamine was not especially widespread or popular, and that great variation existed in patterns of drug use and preferred drugs across specific drug-using scenes.

Jenkins (1994) focused on US media narratives that represented methamphetamine as a new drug (in the form of 'ice' or crystal meth), arguing that the panic they identified was enabled by the existence of another hyperbolic drug-related discourse: that of crack cocaine. In both cases, Jenkins observed, media attention reframed whatever local problems did exist as matters of national significance and these then became the basis for government action (Jenkins 1994, 27).

In a third, more recent, critical sociological analysis, Armstrong (2007) documented the re-emergence of methamphetamine-related 'panic' in the United States, noting its reliance upon an implicit claim that the drug and the issue were both new. Armstrong's paper refined the idea of panic used by Jenkins by drawing on moral panic theory originating in the work of Stanley Cohen (2002 [1972]). It argued that concern about methamphetamine use has been framed in such a way that 'the official reaction to the social condition is out of all proportion to the alleged threat' (Armstrong 2007, 427). Furthermore, Armstrong asserted that the moral panic was aimed explicitly at rural, white, poor people whose economic security had been eroded by global changes in agribusiness, leaving them vulnerable and insufficiently resourced. According to Armstrong, the methamphetamine panic reframed the rural poor as criminal, thereby pre-empting or circumventing broader responsibility for resolving the structural problems they faced.

Following Jenkins and Armstrong, Boyd and Carter (2010) examined the treatment of methamphetamine use in Canadian and US newspapers and other media. They speculated:

> The panicked discourse evident in these news stories suggests that these 'crises' may reflect what David Garland (2008) called an effort to turn methamphetamine use into a 'cultural scapegoat' (p.15) for social anxieties about youth culture, homelessness, and the perceived erosion of racial hierarchies. (2010, 233)

Finally, Ayres and Jewkes (2012) interrogated media images and narratives of a predicted epidemic of crystal meth use in the United Kingdom. They argued that the symbolic, aesthetic and textual representation of crystal meth created its own hyper-reality that bore little relation to the empirical evidence, which suggested that use of the drug was almost non-existent. The alarmist media coverage, which relied heavily on visual images and evidence from the United States, influenced UK political and public debate and drug policy and diverted attention from more urgent social and political issues.

These critical analyses make important arguments about the role of drug discourse in wider political debates and struggles. They help demonstrate that drug research, policy and public discourse are always 'about' other social and political issues. At the same time, they shed light on processes of government. The analysis we present here builds on this work, but departs from it in several ways. First, while ideas of 'panic', including Stanley Cohen's (2002 [1972]) notion of moral panic, have been used to good effect in the critical literature on methamphetamine, we draw instead on recent work in science and technology studies (STS) to examine drug research and policy in a new way. We draw on this work because it makes no claims regarding the 'true' extent of a 'problem' versus the extent implied in the official response to it. In this respect it avoids a major criticism of earlier work on moral panics that accused it of inconsistency in criticising problems as socially constructed while also relying on positivist pronouncements about the 'real' scale of those problems. We also draw on this work because we do not wish to proceed from a claim that the discourse constituting concern about methamphetamine use and those who consume it is homogenous enough to warrant the term 'panic'. Instead, a series of discursive dynamics of rather greater complexity is evident in the material we analyse in this and the next chapter. Finally, unlike these earlier accounts, our specific focus is the relationship between methamphetamine and changing definitions of addiction and dependence.

In this chapter, as in the rest of this book, we look to John Law's work on collateral realities to conduct our analysis, asking the following questions about the enactment of methamphetamine in research accounts:

- What practices – that is, what assemblages of relations – are at work to constitute the realities of methamphetamine use and addiction (here usually termed dependence)?
- How is the stability of these realities achieved and maintained?
- What collateral realities are being done 'incidentally and along the way' (Law 2011, 156) to aid the achievement and maintenance of this stability, and which help to obscure or 'wash away' (Law 2011, 171) this stabilising work?
- What gaps, aporias and tensions exist between these practices and the realities they perform? In other words, which collateral realities might offer entry points for destabilising such accounts?
- Finally, how are articulations of methamphetamine and its collateral realities in these research accounts remaking addiction?

We explore these questions in relation to influential Australian psychological research on the 'amphetamine dependence syndrome' conducted in the 1990s, and documents on 'methamphetamine abuse and addiction' produced by NIDA in the 2000s. The *DSM* and neuroscience we discussed in Chapter 1 are heavily implicated in these two sets of research – the former in Australian attempts to stabilise dependence and the latter in the stabilisation of addiction attempted in the NIDA documents. In Chapter 3, we explore the ways in which methamphetamine addiction is enacted in Australian and US drug policy and in the accounts of those who consume the drug, tracking points of overlap and difference between research, policy and public realities.

Constituting the 'amphetamine dependence syndrome'

The Australian research considers the issue of 'dependence' in relation to 'amphetamine' rather than 'methamphetamine', and therefore requires a brief explanation of terminology. Prior to the late 1990s, amphetamine sulphate was the dominant form of amphetamine in Australian illicit drug markets. From 1998, methamphetamine became the main form of amphetamine available. At approximately the same time as methamphetamine was being identified as an illicit stimulant of concern in Australia, new understandings of stimulants began to emerge that tackled the question of whether the dependence syndrome identified in relation to alcohol and the opiates could be applied to amphetamine. As we show in Chapter 3, while the Australian research dealt with 'amphetamine', the ways in which it produced amphetamine and amphetamine dependence were carried over, and amplified, in relation to methamphetamine. Interestingly, this occurred despite earlier efforts to characterise methamphetamine as distinct from amphetamine. For example, a later Australian report (Topp et al. 2002, 153) notes:

> Although historically the subject of much debate, the existence and destructive nature of a methamphetamine dependence syndrome, comparable to that long acknowledged to exist for alcohol and heroin, was recently documented (Topp & Darke 1997; Topp & Mattick 1997a, b; Topp, Lovibond & Mattick 1998).

Here, the articles cited as documenting the existence of a 'methamphetamine dependence syndrome' all deal specifically with 'amphetamine'. This re-labelling of amphetamine as methamphetamine is widespread (see, for example, McKetin, McLaren & Kelly 2006, 199) and, as we will see, points to a tendency to distinguish the two in accounts emphasising the rise of a new, more potent and more harmful drug – methamphetamine – but to collapse them (usually represented by the term 'meth/amphetamine') in other contexts and for specific strategic purposes (such as when the evidence relating specifically to methamphetamine is limited or unavailable, and to authorise the development of certain policy and practice responses).

How is amphetamine use and dependence constituted in the Australian research, which informed international perceptions of the putative crisis? In this first section we consider the constitutive practices and collateral realities evident in three key research texts: a technical report (Topp et al. 1995) and two journal articles, authored by researchers at Australia's National Drug and Alcohol Research Centre (NDARC) (Topp & Mattick 1997a, b). Published in the late 1990s, these Australian texts aimed to help quantify and respond to an emerging problem by establishing the existence of an amphetamine dependence syndrome and outlining its underlying features. In doing so, they stabilised a version of amphetamine dependence that did not rely on classic formulations of physical withdrawal and tolerance, and played a pivotal role in establishing the reality of an 'amphetamine dependence syndrome'. We have chosen these texts for analysis because the stabilisation of amphetamine dependence they attempted to produce proved influential in subsequent international research and the development of Australian drug policy. For example, the Australian research was cited approvingly as having 'described' a 'clear dependence syndrome' in an Australian government monograph on models of intervention and care for psychostimulant users (Lee 2004, 56). In turn, this monograph became a key part of the evidence base cited in the three Australian policy documents we analyse in the next chapter.

We argue that in these research accounts the stability of amphetamine dependence is achieved and maintained with the aid of the following collateral realities:

- drug policy and practice requires stable objects;
- amphetamine dependence exists (despite extensive critique of the concept from within sociology and psychology);
- dependence is primarily psychological and behavioural rather than physical;
- dependence can occur in non-daily, episodic use, its identifying feature being 'compulsivity'; and
- screening tools provide a sound basis for making important political decisions about the diagnosis of dependent drug use.

The NDARC technical report, and the journal articles that emerged from it, enact several collateral realities in order to stabilise and maintain the object of 'dependence' in general and the 'amphetamine dependence syndrome' in particular. The first collateral reality concerns the overall aim of the publications – to establish a stable object for the purposes of drug policy and practice – and the way in which this aim is expressed bears examination for what it can tell us about the forces in operation in enacting realities of addiction in the context of stimulant use. The technical report begins with a summary of the background to the study. Topp et al. argue that while amphetamine dependence is recognised in 'current psychiatric taxonomies', 'its existence is quite contentious, and little research has examined the applicability of the dependence notions [*sic*] to this drug' (Topp et al. 1995, viii). This 'little [body of] research' focused on amphetamine withdrawal, and drug-taking to relieve withdrawal, as 'hallmarks of amphetamine dependence'. The authors argue:

> These notions fit well with a drug that produces a clearly defined, physiologically based withdrawal syndrome, such as the opiates, but it was *feared* such symptoms may be less relevant to a drug such as amphetamine, for which the withdrawal syndrome is somewhat more *nebulous* [emphasis added]. (1995, viii)

Why should 'fear' be experienced if a syndrome established in relation to alcohol or opiates seems 'less relevant' to amphetamine? The concern here seems to be that existing knowledge might fail in identifying and clarifying a 'nebulous' amphetamine withdrawal syndrome, and dependence more generally. Amphetamine dependence needs to be defined (or, in our terms, enacted as a stable object) if it is to be addressed by policy and practice. Only then can the business of conducting 'research into appropriate interventions for the amphetamine dependence syndrome' (Topp et al. 1995, p. viii) begin.

The second collateral reality made in the technical report concerns past research, namely that it has established a clearly delineated 'dependence syndrome' for alcohol and opiates. This epistemological stance ignores the careful – even tentative – wording evident in sources cited in the report, such as in the proffering of a 'provisional description' of alcohol dependence by psychiatrists Griffith Edwards and Milton Gross (Edwards & Gross 1976). Edwards and Gross explicitly highlight the role of prevailing discourse in shaping understandings of consumption:

> To attempt a definitive description would be premature; much is still only at the stage of 'clinical impression.' *Routine clinical questions may impose a pattern on patients' accounts, and patients themselves organise their uncertain recall of events in terms of expectations given to them.* To link the clinical syndrome with information on the psychobiological basis of dependence is difficult, though scientific understanding has advanced recently. Our aim here is to help further to delineate the clinical picture [emphasis added]. (1976, 1058)

In contrast to Edwards and Gross's 'provisional description' of dependence, the technical report treats it as an uncontroversial, settled concept, and the report's reference list ignores the extensive historical, psychological and sociological debates on the concept that have characterised the field since the late 1970s.[1] It ignores, for example, the existence of two schools of thought on a central and much debated feature of the dependence syndrome. In the first view, Edwards sets forth a traditional view then widely adopted in clinical practice, arguing that at a certain point in their drinking individuals cross an objective divide, regardless of social labels, and become 'dependent':

> We may guess that somewhere within a range of behaviours that go by the name of alcoholism, there lies a condition which is not to be understood in terms of variation but rather in terms of state. We try today to catch its image descriptively in terms of the dependence syndrome while others before us have certainly been trying to perceive its outline in terms of 'alcoholism as a disease'. We are guessing though that somewhere in that landscape there is a real beast to be described rather than an arbitrary cut on a continuum, a label, an abominable and mythical medicalisation. (1980, 309)

Once an individual becomes dependent, signalled by this change in psychobiological state, the level of dependence can be classified according to degree.[2]

A second school of thought, what we might call the continuum model, views dependence on any activity or substance as normal rather than pathological. All individuals can be placed on the continuum of dependence, which ranges from 'nil' through 'mild' and 'moderate' to 'severe'. For those espousing this more psychological perspective (such as Russell [1976] and Orford [1985]), alcohol dependence was a question of variation rather than a discrete state. The two schools of thought, while differing on this important point, shared an explicit focus on individual behaviour while allowing for social, cultural and economic factors in the 'colouring' of the syndrome.

Other researchers, many of whom sought to emphasise the historical, social and cultural contexts of alcohol and other drug use, were more critical. They argued that 'alcohol dependence' was merely the 'disease' model repackaged and rejuvenated for the 1980s, a means of neutering sustained challenges to the medical field from disciplines such as psychology and sociology. Shaw (1979), for example, argued that the WHO's speedy adoption of what had been described by Edwards and Gross as a 'provisional syndrome' in the ninth edition of its *International Classification of Diseases* (1979) lent weight to the view that political motives, rather than scientific ones, underlay its ready acceptance.

In a later publication, he (Shaw 1985, 41) questioned the terms of the syndrome again, arguing:

> It seems plain to me . . . that factors extraneous to those included in the framework of the dependence syndrome must actually be more important in determining the natural history of a drinking career.

Some chose a more cautious middle position, arguing that the syndrome provided a coherent description of a particular type of alcohol use but that more research was required (Thorley 1985), or attempted to refine the concept (Hodgson & Stockwell 1985). Still others differentiated between the social and cultural aspects of alcohol and other drug dependence and those of a physical nature and argued that the interrelation between them was determined by the prevailing social and cultural contexts of use (Room 1987; Moore 1992) argued that in spite of its medical setting the concept retained its moral underpinnings and that its diagnostic criteria remained ambiguous. These criticisms and discussions of dependence, all of which were available in the published literature, are absent from the Australian texts, which deliver a noticeably narrow account of the development and acceptance of the concept.

The third collateral reality enacted in the Australian account of amphetamine dependence is that dependence is primarily psychological and behavioural rather than physical. The authors approvingly cite an earlier attempt (Edwards et al. 1984) to broaden the application of the 'dependence syndrome' to take in other drugs such as amphetamine. In their view (Topp et al. 1995, viii), this broadening of the concept

> *reduced the traditional emphasis* [in the original formulation of dependence on alcohol] on tolerance and withdrawal, and *attached greater importance* to symptoms of a compulsion to use, a narrowing of the drug-using repertoire, rapid reinstatement of dependence after abstinence, and the high salience of drug use in the user's life [emphasis added].

Yet, it is not clear from a close reading of Edwards et al. (1984) that in the move from alcohol to a consideration of other drugs there is indeed a 'reduced' emphasis on tolerance and withdrawal nor that 'greater importance' has been attached to the psychological and behavioural aspects of dependence. The authors list seven 'cognitive, behavioural, and physiological' 'phenomena or dimensions' of dependence that can be used to identify its existence without ranking or prioritising their importance: subjective awareness of a compulsion to use drugs, a desire to cease drug use, narrowing of behavioural repertoire, tolerance and withdrawal symptoms, relief from or avoidance of withdrawal symptoms through drug use, salience of drug use and rapid reinstatement of dependence following abstinence. They (Edwards et al. 1984, 82) explicitly state:

> Although the model [of dependence] displays what we believe to be many of the relevant phenomena and their many connexions, we are not able to state a degree of significance or weighting to be given to any particular factor or connexion.

The equal weighting of the seven criteria in this formulation was also echoed in the *DSM-IIIR* and *DSM-IV* (although the *DSM* categories did not replicate the alcohol dependence criteria exactly).

So far, we have identified the constitution of three collateral realities of amphetamine dependence in the NDARC technical report: it must be defined for policy and practice, and as such it is enacted as a stable object; it constitutes a definite syndrome; and it does not need to entail physical tolerance and withdrawal. Having established amphetamine dependence in this way, Topp et al. then go on to state the twin aims of their research:

> [T]o determine, firstly, whether there *is* an amphetamine dependence syndrome, and secondly, to begin explicating what the dimensions underlying such a syndrome might be ... (1995, viii)

The first aim of establishing the existence of the amphetamine dependence syndrome seems somewhat pre-ordained by their need to define amphetamine dependence for policy and practical purposes. It also seems somewhat circular because the 132 'regular amphetamine users' who were the subjects of the study had already been defined as 'dependent [on amphetamine] by *DSM-III-R* criteria'. Their second aim – to delineate the dimensions underlying the syndrome – also takes for granted that the syndrome exists. Finally, their idiosyncratic reading of Edwards et al.'s 1984 article had already de-emphasised tolerance and withdrawal in favour of psychological and behavioural aspects, thus allowing the incorporation of amphetamine into dependence.

The collateral realities enacted in the technical report are reinforced in the two journal articles that emerged from it. In the first article, Topp and Mattick (1997a) attempt to validate the existence of an amphetamine dependence syndrome using the Severity of Amphetamine Dependence Questionnaire (SAmDQ). As its name suggests, the SAmDQ is a clinical and research tool for measuring the severity of amphetamine dependence; it was adapted from the Severity of Opiate Dependence Questionnaire (Churchill et al. 1993). Like the technical report, the article begins with an outline of the broadening of the original dependence syndrome to include drugs other than alcohol and opiates. The authors (Topp & Mattick) state that the newer version of the dependence syndrome

> retained the emphasis of the disease model of addiction on tolerance and withdrawal, but in conceptualizing a *dimension* of severity of dependence, also attached greater importance to symptoms such as a compulsion to use, a narrowing of the drug-using repertoire, rapid reinstatement of dependence after abstinence, and the high salience of drug use in the user's life. (1997a, 151)

This explanation introduces two terms that muddy the conceptual waters of addiction: disease and dimension. While 'disease' describes a categorical condition characterised by physical tolerance and withdrawal, 'dimension' has slightly different meanings (*OED* online version, accessed 2 August 13): '1. a measurable extent of a particular kind, such as length, breadth, depth, or height…2. an aspect or feature of a situation'. In other words, whereas addiction as disease is categorical, dependence as dimension relates to both category and continuum. Here, the authors combine two apparently incompatible ontological framings of dependence – as categorical disease and as continuum – under the same term.[3]

What strategic benefits might accrue from adding the framing of amphetamine dependence as continuum to the existing framing of dependence as category, and from emphasising the psychological and behavioural aspects of dependence? What collateral reality of addiction is being produced in these moves? An answer becomes apparent when we come to the discussion section of the article. Here, the authors argue that their findings suggest that amphetamine dependence shares many similarities with opiate dependence and 'support the existence of a dependence construct that is comprised of [*sic*] physical and affective withdrawal and withdrawal relief drug-taking' (Topp & Mattick 1997a, 160). However, they also note that although the

> dependence syndrome comprised of [sic] these underlying dimensions is manifest in those amphetamine users who administer the drug virtually every day... many surveys [and indeed their own research] indicate that these users are in the minority. Individuals can manifest dangerous patterns of stimulant use that *do not* include daily administration and, if the withdrawal and withdrawal relief symptoms assessed in the SAmDQ are considered the hallmarks of amphetamine dependence, then it is possible that the severity of dependence of these users could be underestimated. (1997a, 160)

In this conclusion, we see a fourth collateral reality being enacted to achieve and maintain the stability of the amphetamine dependence syndrome: 'binge' consumption patterns as 'dependence'. This remaking of dependence itself helps stabilise the reality of the amphetamine dependence syndrome in that it allows greater numbers of people – many of whose consumption patterns do not have the regularity once considered the hallmark of dependence – to be pathologised as dependent. In order to explain this difference, Topp and Mattick suggest that further research is needed on

> symptoms of a compulsion to use [which is not defined] and salience of drug use in the user's life... in order to assess the level of dependence of these individuals who, while less dependent than daily users, still manifest problematic patterns of use [also not defined]. (1997a, 160)

Here, dependence is extended to a wider range of drug use practices and has come to be characterised by fine-grained but poorly articulated distinctions.

In the second journal article (Topp & Mattick 1997b), we see the final collateral reality referred to in the introduction to this section being mobilised to achieve and maintain the stable object of amphetamine dependence – that screening tools allow us to identify and measure dependence reliably, and in doing so, make possible important political decisions regarding the diagnosis of dependent drug use. Topp and Mattick aim to develop a cut-off score on the Severity of Dependence Scale (SDS) which would indicate 'clinically significant amphetamine dependence'. The SDS, like the SAmDQ, evolved from an opiate-specific clinical and research instrument (the Opiate Subjective Dependence Questionnaire) and was designed to measure dependence on drugs other than opiates (Gossop et al. 1992). In Topp and Mattick's (1997b, 840) view, the value of the SDS 'as a measure of dependence arises from its comprehensibility and ease of administration'. The article's Introduction ignores the role of measurement practices in constituting research objects (such as 'dependence') and again invokes some of the collateral realities we identified earlier: that dependence exists and that it need not entail physical tolerance and withdrawal.

The SDS involves the administration of five questions (cited in Topp & Mattick 1997b, 841):

(1) Did you think your use of [amphetamine] was out of control?
(2) Did the prospect of missing a hit (line, dose) make you very anxious or worried?
(3) Did you worry about your use of [amphetamine]?
(4) Did you wish you could stop?
(5) How difficult would you find it to stop or go without [amphetamine]?

These questions focus on the qualities and capacities held to be central to neo-liberal subjects: self-regulation, independence and autonomy (Moore & Fraser 2006). Topp and Mattick's rationale for using the SDS rather than the *DSM-III-R* and for 'choosing' an SDS cut-off score relate to the requirements of clinical assessment. Whereas the *DSM-III-R* takes approximately 40 minutes to administer, the SDS can be administered in less than a minute. Therefore, if the SDS provides a reasonable indication of dependence, then it can 'potentially be used as a screening instrument to identify individuals with problematic patterns of drug use who require further assessment' (Topp & Mattick 1997b, 840). The *DSM* is, in Topp and Mattick's view, more reliable and comprehensive but takes too long to administer. By contrast, the SDS had 'high diagnostic utility' because its ease of use trumps its lack of 'sensitivity and specificity' (Topp & Mattick 1997b, 839).

Although, as already noted, Topp and Mattick approvingly cite earlier work that moved away from a categorical approach to dependence to one that emphasised dimension (that is, continuum), they reinstate the categorical emphasis in their analysis:

> For the purposes of this analysis, which requires that there be only two levels of the 'gold standard' variable (in medical terminology, 'disease present' or 'case' and 'disease absent' or 'non-case'), the sample was divided into two groups on the basis of the *DSM-III-R*

> diagnosis derived from the CIDI [Composite International Diagnostic Interview – the WHO's mental health screening tool]. (1997b, 841)

Thus, their aim is to create a dichotomy between those who are dependent on amphetamine and those who are not. Such a categorical emphasis is at odds with the position outlined in Edwards et al.'s article approvingly cited by Topp and Mattick and which provides the overall inspiration for their study. In it, Edwards et al. state:

> The dependence syndrome is not absolute, but is a quantitative phenomenon that exists in different degrees... On the basis of current knowledge, *no sharp cut-off point can be identified for distinguishing drug dependence from non-dependent but recurrent drug use* [emphasis added]. (1984, 80)

The political stakes in these mechanisms for ascribing dependence states are extremely high. Although the SDS is designed to 'identify individuals with problematic patterns of use', its questions focus on subjective self-assessment of individual psychological states rather than patterns of drug use or the problems arising from use. Furthermore, the instrument used to categorise drug users as dependent or non-dependent takes less than a minute to administer. It is no exaggeration to say the ascription of the label 'dependent' is an important social decision concerning the creation, classification and management of drug-using subjects: it informs policy as well as public perceptions of drug problems via media reporting of research findings. It also has serious personal consequences for those individuals so designated. In a social and cultural context in which neo-liberal discourse valorises self-regulation, independence and closely allied capacities such as rationality and responsibility, being categorised as dependent carries heavy costs; it enacts individuals as potentially 'failed' citizens and subjects (Keane 2002; Moore & Fraser 2006). Even if we accept the need for such classification in the case of amphetamine, where to then? When Topp and Mattick's article was published, few treatments for amphetamine dependence were available (an issue we take up more fully in Chapter 3). It therefore remains unclear how the application of the cut-off score in the SDS – how, that is, the enactment of the reality of amphetamine dependence via five brief questions that take neo-liberal autonomy and rationality for granted – improves the standing and well-being of drug users.

So far in this chapter we have examined the collateral realities enacted in the constitution of amphetamine use and dependence in three

Australian research texts. First, we identified an epistemological 'fear': that existing research had so far failed to stabilise a 'nebulous' and 'contentious' amphetamine withdrawal syndrome to allow the development and implementation of policy and provision of services. Second, we traced how dependence was enacted in these research texts as clearly delineated, settled and uncontroversial rather than 'provisional', despite extensive critique and in the absence of any consideration of historical, social and cultural context. Third, we saw how dependence was remade as primarily psychological and behavioural rather than physical. This prioritising of specific diagnostic criteria was directly at odds with Edwards et al.'s (1984) original work on dependence, which is cited by the Australian texts, and also at odds with the *DSM-IIIR* and *DSM-IV*. Fourth, we observed the process by which dependence was remade into a broader assemblage that included non-daily, episodic use. With the shift in emphasis from physical tolerance and withdrawal, the primary subject of dependence became the 'compulsive' (that is, pathological) drug user. Finally, we showed how, with amphetamine dependence stabilised, attention turned to devising a convenient screening tool and cut-off score for 'clinically significant amphetamine dependence'. This quietly reinstated categorical disease-present/disease-absent binary, and the SDS's focus on neo-liberal attributes, became the basis for important political decisions regarding the creation, classification and management of dependent drug users.

Some of the issues we have identified in the Australian texts, which played a significant role in establishing the reality of an 'amphetamine dependence syndrome' and subsequently influenced international research and Australian drug policy, emerge in other contexts in which amphetamine and methamphetamine are discussed. In the next section, we analyse documents on methamphetamine produced in the 2000s in the United States by NIDA. Although there are continuities and similarities between the Australian publications of the 1990s and the NIDA publications of the 2000s, a key difference is the rise of neuroscientific accounts of addiction in NIDA publications on methamphetamine and other drugs.

Making methamphetamine in the United States and beyond

In this section, we analyse the collateral realities at work in two versions of the NIDA publication *Methamphetamine Abuse and Addiction*, part of its *Research Report Series*. The first version was originally published in 1998 and reprinted in 2002 (NIDA 2002); the second version was revised and published in 2006 (NIDA 2006a). Although we focus mainly on these two publications and some of the key differences between them, the ways in which they enact the realities of methamphetamine use and 'addiction', the drug's effect on the brain, the scale of methamphetamine 'abuse', and the characteristics of those who consume methamphetamine and of the drug itself are evident in a range of other NIDA publications on methamphetamine (for example, NIDA 2006b, 2010a) and on 'drug abuse' more generally (for example, NIDA 2010b). We acknowledge that these and other NIDA publications are produced within (and perhaps for) the US policy context, which has long been out of step with many other Western countries, but there are good reasons to treat them as key sites in the constitution of drug-related realities. Their easy availability on the NIDA website means that they are freely accessible to an international audience, and NIDA funds approximately 86% of the world's research on drugs (Courtwright 2010). NIDA's scientific authority and US drug policy also exert significant influence over international research, policy settings and regulatory frameworks, treaties and laws.

We argue that the NIDA documents work to constitute and stabilise the realities of methamphetamine abuse and addiction through the following collateral realities (most of which are also in operation in the Australian texts already analysed):

- methamphetamine is a growing problem and highly addictive;
- methamphetamine addiction is the outcome of biological changes;
- science (especially neuroscience and surveillance research) delivers undisputed facts;
- there is a clear relationship between methamphetamine and harm; and
- treatments for methamphetamine addiction are available.

In 2002, NIDA released an updated, second version of *Methamphetamine Abuse and Addiction*, its key text on the subject of methamphetamine. Comprising seven pages, it uses text, boxes, images and tables, and concludes with a Glossary and Resources section. The 'serious' and 'alarming' nature of the topic covered by the report is immediately signalled by the formatting of its title, with 'methamphetamine' set in bolded and shadowed capitals and 'abuse and addiction' italicised and shadowed. These design features (the functions of which are also analysed, at a general level, by John Law [2011]) vividly suggest coverage of a sinister topic, contrasting sharply with the rest of the document, which is set out in typically bland report style.

The cover page of the 2002 report introduces the first collateral reality referred to above: methamphetamine is highly addictive, and its use is a growing problem. It features an introductory message from Dr Glen A. Hanson, NIDA's Acting Director, which begins by describing methamphetamine as a 'potent' psychostimulant and its 'abuse' as an 'extremely serious and growing problem'. Later, Hanson refers to 'dramatic increases in its use' alongside a bar graph depicting emergency department mentions of methamphetamine from 1997 to 2000. Two discursive strategies are immediately apparent in the text. First, in his opening sentences, Hanson makes no distinction between 'abuse' and 'use'. This is a general feature of the document about which we say more below. Second, the bar graph does not support his assertion that the problem is 'growing', at least as it refers to methamphetamine. The graph shows that methamphetamine mentions decreased from approximately 17,000 to approximately 13,000, although amphetamine mentions increased from approximately 10,000 to approximately 16,000. This might seem a minor quibble until one considers how methamphetamine is contrasted with amphetamine in the report. Although methamphetamine's 'chemical structure' is described as 'similar to that of amphetamine', its effects on the central nervous system are described as 'more pronounced'.

We see similar statements in the NIDA Director's message that opens the 2006 edition of the report. Like Hanson before her, the new director Dr Nora D. Volkow describes methamphetamine as 'highly addictive' and uses statistics to support her claim that its 'abuse continues to spread', and is 'increasingly' affecting both rural and urban areas. However, rather like Hanson's puzzling use of the graph, she cites research that cannot prove her point: a cross-sectional survey on lifetime use rather than a longitudinal study.

The second collateral reality enacted in these reports is that addiction is biological. Given the claim that methamphetamine is highly addictive, how is addiction to methamphetamine defined in the NIDA documents and how is it distinguished from other patterns of consumption? Although both documents use the terms 'addiction' and 'abuse' in their titles, nowhere is the difference between the two categories, or what is meant by 'abuse', defined. Furthermore, throughout the documents, the term 'use', also undefined, is used interchangeably with 'abuse' and 'addiction' in confusing and contradictory ways; both use and abuse are further qualified with the adjective 'chronic', also without definition.

For example, 'abuse' is deployed in discussing surveys of lifetime use (in which at least some of the reported consumption must, by definition, be at very low levels), but 'use' is deployed in discussing the binge pattern (NIDA 2002, 3) said to characterise methamphetamine addiction.

The reader must wait until page 4 (2002) and page 5 (2006a) of the reports before addiction is defined: 'Addiction is a chronic, relapsing disease, characterized by compulsive drug-seeking and drug use which is accompanied by functional and molecular changes in the brain.'[4] This definition immediately prompts several questions. What exactly is meant by 'accompanied by'? Is the disease of addiction absent if scans and other forms of technology cannot detect functional and molecular changes in the brain? If these functional and molecular changes in the brain are present in the brain scans, can addiction be diagnosed by recourse to the scans alone? Do brain images therefore make addiction?

Later, the document states:

> Although there are no physical manifestations of a withdrawal syndrome when methamphetamine use is stopped, there are several symptoms that occur when a chronic user stops taking the drug. These include depression, anxiety, fatigue [which seems at least partly physical], paranoia, aggression, and an intense craving for the drug.
>
> (NIDA 2002, 5)

Importantly, at least three of the symptoms listed as arising from the cessation of methamphetamine – paranoia, aggression and craving – also appear in the descriptions of typical behaviour when using the drug. The symptoms, it seems, are caused by both the presence *and* absence of methamphetamine.

This enactment of addiction is also significant for the way it positions episodic patterns of use. In its focus on chronicity and compulsion, it echoes long-standing definitions of alcohol and heroin addiction. Yet, as with the Australian publications discussed earlier, the NIDA documents depart radically from such definitions when they state that methamphetamine is most often used in a binge pattern. Along with this departure, and contrary to orthodox understandings of tolerance as the need to use larger amounts of a drug over time to produce the same effect,[5] the 2002 report treats tolerance in a new and unique way:

> Because tolerance for methamphetamine occurs *within minutes* – meaning that the pleasurable effects disappear even before the drug

> concentration in the blood falls significantly – users try to maintain the high by binging [*sic*] on the drug [emphasis added].[6]
>
> (NIDA 2002, 3)

Here, in the absence of 'physical manifestations of a withdrawal syndrome', and faced with explaining an episodic pattern of use that does not progress to a daily pattern of use (as NIDA has long warned is a danger of drug use in general), the 2002 report is compelled to generate a new definition of an existing phenomenon – tolerance. Whereas the Australian publications deploy psychological dysfunction through their use of the pathologising and undefined term 'compulsion' to explain this, the NIDA reports resort to a biological explanation that relies on an unprecedented and idiosyncratic definition of tolerance (and one which they abandon in later pages).

Both Hanson (in the 2002 report) and Volkow (in the 2006 report) identify their main aim as 'provid[ing] an overview of the latest scientific findings' on methamphetamine. In both editions of the report, this overview is limited to neuroscience and surveillance research on drug trends. Here we see the first instance of the third collateral reality referred to above, that of science – even when represented by a very narrow range of studies (and particularly neuroscience, in which NIDA has invested heavily) – as allowing access to unalloyed truth. Volkow provides a particularly stark example of advocacy for the enlightening and progressive potential of science when she writes, in her foreword to *Drugs, Brains, and Behavior: The Science of Addiction*:

> Throughout much of the last century, scientists studying drug abuse labored in the shadows of powerful myths and misconceptions about the nature of addiction . . . Today, thanks to science, our views and responses to drug abuse have changed dramatically. Groundbreaking discoveries about the brain have revolutionized our understanding of drug addiction, enabling us to respond effectively to the problem.
>
> (NIDA 2010b, 1)

The reality of science as indisputable, and as monolithic, is enacted in the text in part by a departure from research referencing conventions. With the exception of tables, and the brain images we discuss below, no references are cited at the appropriate points in the text to support specific claims. Instead, they are merely listed under a 'Resources' subheading ('References' in the 2006 version) at the end of the report. This textual strategy makes it difficult to check the original sources to verify the specific claims they are mobilised to support. One could hardly find a more explicit strategy of 'washing away' the stabilising work done by the collateral reality of 'science'.

As we have noted, key statements regarding methamphetamine rely heavily on the authority of neuroscience. For example, methamphetamine's toxic effects on the brain are established by reference to animal studies, in which

> a single high dose of the drug has been shown to damage nerve terminals in the dopamine-containing regions of the brain. The large release of dopamine produced by methamphetamine is thought to contribute to the drug's toxic effects on nerve terminals in the brain.
>
> (NIDA 2002, 4)

Animal studies are also referenced in the section on long-term effects, again in relation to the neurotoxic effects of methamphetamine:

> In scientific studies examining the consequences of long-term methamphetamine exposure in animals, concern has arisen over its toxic effects on the brain. Researchers have reported that as much as 50 per cent of the dopamine-producing cells in the brain can be damaged after prolonged exposure to relatively low levels of methamphetamine.
>
> (NIDA 2002, 5)

The weaknesses of such claims are well known, the most relevant here being uncertainty about whether the doses administered in research on animals bear any resemblance to those typically consumed by humans (Hart et al. 2012). The relevance of such research is thrown further into doubt by the admission that '[w]hether this [neuro]toxicity is related to the psychosis seen in some long-term methamphetamine abusers is still an open question' (NIDA 2002, 5).

The stabilising work being done by the collateral reality of neuroscience in both reports also consists of visual images of the brain (see also Chapter 1). For example, the 2006 edition includes a boxed set of three brain scans (taken from NIDA Director Nora Volkow's own research). The box is titled 'Recovery of Brain Dopamine Transporters in Chronic Methamphetamine (METH) Abusers'. Under the title are representations of three brains: one is captioned 'Normal Control', the second 'METH Abuser (1 month abstinence)' and the third 'METH Abuser (24 month abstinence)'. The box stands entirely alone in the report. The pictured brains certainly look different from one another, but there are no instructions on how to interpret these differences. No reference is made in the main text to 'transporters', and dopamine is discussed only in general terms in relation to its function in the brain and the impairment of its re-uptake by methamphetamine. In other words, it is impossible to make sense of the images. What is their purpose? What do they mean? That 'METH abusers' are not 'normal'? That the 'addicted subject' should be defined primarily by (uninterpretable) changes in the brain? Or that the reader should rest assured in the knowledge that neuroscience has the answers?

Latour's (2004) critique of the realist ontological hierarchy between 'primary' (that is, objective) and 'secondary [i.e. subjective] qualities' offers a useful way of thinking critically about the use of brain scans in NIDA documents and elsewhere. He notes that under the 'modernist predicament' any discussion of the body seems inevitably to lead to physiology and medicine, and to the idea that a reductionist science can progressively reveal the body's primary qualities (such as the structures and DNA sequences of brains and neurons).[7] Other versions of what it is to be a body – for example, subjective embodiment and other aspects that are seen to 'exist only in our minds, imaginations and cultural accounts' (Latour 2004, 208) – are relegated to the sphere of secondary qualities. Furthermore (Latour 2004, 224), adopting this 'eliminativist' view means that '[o]nce we have a way of grasping the primary qualities [of the body] ... we can eliminate as irrelevant all other versions of what it is to be a body, that is, to be somebody'.

Latour proposes a different approach to these issues. Rather than seeing the biomedical articulations of the body as reductionist, primary and objective, he offers a science studies perspective:

> There is no primary quality, no scientist can be reductionist, disciplines can only *add* to the world and almost never subtract phenomena . . . Reductionism is not a sin for which scientists should make amends, but a dream precisely as unreachable as being alive and having *no* body.
>
> (Latour 2004, 226)

Applying Latour's argument, we can argue that the authority of the NIDA scans of the brains of 'METH abusers' derives from biomedicine's ontological politics – that is, from its modernist claim to possess unmediated access to an objective material world of primary qualities that are fundamentally responsible for health, life and social existence, and that with work, knowledge can be distilled such that this objective world can be discovered. In Latour's view, if other versions of the body are to be sustained in the face of bio-industry's expansion into 'all the details of our daily existence' (for example, versions of the body articulated by drug consumers), then we cannot agree to 'give science the imperial right of defining all by itself the entire realm of primary qualities, while militancy limits itself to the residual province of subjective feelings' (Latour 2004, 227).

Of course, dissenting views regarding the relationship between methamphetamine use and brain function can also be found within neuroscience. These, however, rely upon the same ontological and epistemological assumptions as the collateral reality of neuroscience enacted in the NIDA documents. For example, in 2012, Carl Hart and colleagues published a critical article (Hart et al. 2012) in *Neuropsychopharmacology*, the journal of the American College of Neuropsychopharmacology.[8] This review of the published literature on methamphetamine use and cognitive deficit focuses on the acute and long-term effects of methamphetamine, and assesses the contribution of brain-imaging studies to illuminating the neural mechanisms underlying methamphetamine's effects on cognitive function. They conclude that the data on acute effects show that 'methamphetamine improves cognitive performance of both methamphetamine abusers and non-users in some domains, for example, visuospatial perception, sustained attention, and response speed, even when larger intranasal and intravenous doses are tested' (Hart et al. 2012, 604). Conversely, 'methamphetamine-induced disruptive cognitive effects were not observed and therefore rarely reported' (Hart et al. 2012, 604). Although neural differences between methamphetamine users and control participants have been reported in various studies, there have been 'few replications of specific findings' (2012, 604). Hart et al. (2012, 604) suggest that these findings 'might be spurious and unrelated to methamphetamine use'. The studies also typically employed limited cognitive measures and often found that the 'cognitive functioning of methamphetamine users generally fell within the normal range' (2012, 604). Despite these problems, 'researchers frequently interpreted any brain differences as indicative of cognitive pathologies caused by the abuse of methamphetamine' (2012, 604).

In their discussion of the implications of their critical review, Hart et al. raise several issues. First, they suggest that researchers need to re-evaluate their starting assumption that methamphetamine causes cognitive impairment because this has unduly shaped the interpretation of research findings. Second, they find little evidence to support the not-uncommon view that methamphetamine-related cognitive impairments might compromise the ability to engage in treatment. Third, they argue that public policy on methamphetamine should be less drastic and punitive because of the high monetary and human costs. They close with the following observation:

> Many of the claims about methamphetamine-associated cognitive impairments are reminiscent of statements made about crack cocaine more than two decades ago before the empirical evidence was clear. Taken together, these observations lead us to speculate whether we are headed down this path once again.
>
> (Hart et al. 2012, 605)

Despite their criticism of existing neuroscience research on methamphetamine use and cognitive deficit, including the research of NIDA Director Nora Volkow, and despite their observation that preconceptions can shape data analysis (or, as we might put it, data is not independent of interpretation – realities are made in practice), Hart and his colleagues remain very much wedded to the neuroscience paradigm. Rather like the Australian studies, which ignore the role of measurement practices in constituting research objects (such as 'dependence'), they treat cognitive deficits in the brains of methamphetamine users as ontologically anterior to, and independent of, scientific attempts to identify them. They imply that it is possible to identify and document these deficits using established scientific methods and epistemology. Thus their criticisms of faulty interpretation and insufficient evidence emerge from the same ontological and epistemological grounds as the science they criticise – their critique is thus primarily a call for better research of the same type.

In addition to neuroscience, the NIDA documents rely on surveillance research to establish patterns of methamphetamine use and, in doing so, introduce as many questions as does the neuroscience. For example, the section on the 'scope of methamphetamine abuse' in the 2006 report contains some important contradictions. Following opening claims that methamphetamine *abuse* is spreading across the country and growing in scale, it presents cross-sectional survey data on the lifetime, past-year and current prevalence of *use* from the 2005 National Survey on Drug Use and Health, and data on the lifetime prevalence of *use* from the Monitoring the Future survey of secondary school students conducted in the same year. According to the report, both surveys show *declines* in 'methamphetamine abuse' (remembering that definitions of what constitutes 'use' and 'abuse' have not been provided).

The next three paragraphs of the 2006 report consider emergency department (ED) statistics from the Drug Abuse Warning Network and data on treatment admissions. The former show a greater than 50% increase in the 'number of ED visits related to methamphetamine abuse' between 1995 and 2002 while statistics on treatment admissions for methamphetamine abuse 'have also increased substantially', rising from 1 to 8% of all admissions between 1992 and 2004 – a trend that is 'spreading across the country'. Two points are worth noting here. First, the statistics presented cover treatment admissions in which methamphetamine or amphetamine were 'identified as the primary drug of abuse' – thus, we again see the conflation of amphetamine with its supposedly more potent derivative, methamphetamine. Second, in the close alignment of ED data on the acute outcomes of episodic methamphetamine use with data on treatment admissions (which presumably relate to methamphetamine 'addiction'), we can again discern the expansion of addiction to include a binge pattern of compulsive use. Here addiction is made not as a chronic pattern of daily use leading to physical withdrawal on cessation, but, at least partly, as relating to bingeing or other unacceptable patterns of consumption. It seems that although NIDA enacts science – epidemiology as well as neuroscience – as an indisputable source of transparent facts about the world, the slipperiness, ambiguity and partiality of these facts is never far from view.

A final observation about NIDA's reliance on the collateral reality of science as undisputed fact is that, in both versions of the report, and in *Drugs, Brains, and Behavior* (NIDA 2010b), reference to the substantial body of qualitative research on the social contexts and cultural meanings of methamphetamine use is entirely absent. This absence becomes particularly germane when we reach the section on methamphetamine 'use' in the 2002 version ('abuse' in the 2006 version), in which readers are informed that the drug 'alters moods in different ways, depending on how it is taken' (2002, 3). In both versions, this leads to a discussion of modes of consuming methamphetamine. Smoking or injecting the drug produces 'an intense rush or "flash" that lasts only a few minutes and is described as extremely pleasurable' (note the distancing effect of the caveat 'is described as', as though the experiences and opinions of methamphetamine consumers should be treated cautiously while, later in the reports, the neuroscience of pleasure is described extensively). Snorting or swallowing methamphetamine produces 'euphoria – a high but not an intense rush'. This concentration on mode of ingestion as the exclusive shaper of drug-related experiences ignores the large body of social research on the importance of the cultural, social and historical contexts of drug use (for just a few examples, see Becker 1963; MacAndrew & Edgerton 1969; Levine 1978; Zinberg 1984; Gomart 2002, 2004). In this way, the complex phenomenon of methamphetamine use – which emerges from assemblages of substance, bodies, emotions, and human and non-human actors – is over-simplified in the interests of stabilisation.

A similar strategic erasure of qualitative research from the collateral reality of science enacted by NIDA occurs in the first section of the 2002 report's main text, which is subheaded 'What is methamphetamine?' This section opens with vivid prose describing methamphetamine as a 'powerfully addictive stimulant that dramatically affects the central nervous system' (1). The text goes on to note the ease with which methamphetamine can be manufactured and this, combined with its addictive power, 'make[s] methamphetamine a drug with high potential for widespread abuse'. As we have already noted, the international literature on the social context, cultural meanings and political economy of drug use is given no part in this account, in which supply and pharmacology take the primary causal roles. Indeed, no consideration is given to demand for methamphetamine, and the vast differences in cultures and patterns of methamphetamine use between clubbers (sometimes in combination with 'club' or 'party' drugs) (Duff 2005); gay men (Clatts et al. 2001; Slavin 2004; Halkitis et al. 2005); injecting drug users (Zule & Desmond 1999) and ethnic groups (Joe 1996; Brown 2010). Nor does it admit the possibility of 'functional' methamphetamine use (Lende et al. 2007). Here, the 'social' is erased and with it also the need to address issues of race, class, gender, inequality and marginalisation. The focus on supply and pharmacology sits comfortably with an emphasis on law enforcement and treatment responses.

A fourth collateral reality enacted in the NIDA publications is that there is a clear relationship between methamphetamine and harm. In Hanson's message in the 2002 report, he states that methamphetamine is a 'powerfully addictive stimulant associated with serious health conditions' (NIDA 2002, 1). Yet, in the main body of the document, the relationship between methamphetamine consumption and various forms of harm, already described rather vaguely by Hanson as an 'association', is further diluted and confused. For example, methamphetamine 'may', 'can' and is 'thought to contribute to' a range of short- and long-term effects. The boxed text listing 'short-term effects' conflates aspects of the methamphetamine experience that, according to a large body of international qualitative research, drug consumers actively seek (such as 'increased attention and decreased fatigue', 'euphoria and rush'), with those that might be seen as forms of harm (such as 'hyperthermia'). The treatment of long-term effects in the report is much less equivocal, which is in keeping with its general tone: 'Long-term methamphetamine abuse results in many damaging effects, including addiction' (4).

In the 2002 edition of the report, Hanson also draws attention to NIDA's goal of translating research so as to 'develop more effective strategies for [the] prevention and treatment' of 'drug abuse and addiction' (NIDA 2002, 1). Here we see a fifth collateral reality at work: that effective treatments exist for methamphetamine addiction. This collateral reality is also evident in the 2006 edition of the report and, as we highlighted above, in other NIDA publications such as *Drugs, Brains, and Behavior* (NIDA 2010b). Significantly, by the time we reach the section on treatment, neuroscience is nowhere to be found. Instead we are informed that the 'most effective treatments for methamphetamine addiction are cognitive behavioral interventions' (2002, 6). These interventions encourage the realisation of a self-moderating, neo-liberal subject through their focus on helping to 'modify the patient's thinking, expectancies, and behaviors and to increase skills in coping with various life stressors' (2002, 6) (one might wonder if these 'life stressors' include the absence of a welfare safety net and a living wage). As David Courtwright (2010) has noted, NIDA's significant financial investment in and championing of the 'brain disease paradigm' has not led to more effective treatment strategies but back to cognitive behavioural therapy (CBT), an approach that first emerged in the 1960s – well before brain imaging, neurotransmitters, synapses and neural reward systems were implicated in understandings of addiction.

In summary, in the texts examined above NIDA enacts several collateral realities in its attempts to stabilise methamphetamine addiction. First, the texts produce methamphetamine as highly agential, as an 'addictive', 'potent' stimulant whose 'abuse' is an 'extremely serious and growing problem'. This is achieved by confusing 'abuse' and 'use', conflating amphetamine and methamphetamine, and drawing on cross-sectional rather than longitudinal data. Second, they invoke a binge pattern of use as characteristic of methamphetamine addiction and, in the absence of evidence for physical withdrawal, resort to an unprecedented and idiosyncratic definition of tolerance to explain compulsive use and addiction as biological. Third, they expand addiction to include bingeing and other forms of heavy episodic consumption by treating neuroscience and surveillance research as undisputed fact. In deploying brain scans that are uninterpretable (because of the absence of explanatory text or captions), they rely heavily on biomedicine's ontological politics to claim unmediated access to an objective material world of primary qualities. They also misrepresent statistical data on methamphetamine use, ED visits and treatment admissions. In ignoring the international literature on the contexts of methamphetamine use, they erase the 'social' and the need to address race, class, gender, inequality and marginalisation in understanding drug use. Fourth, the texts fudge the relationship between methamphetamine and harm, describing it variously as an association, a possible contribution and a definite cause. Finally, despite lauding the promise of neuroscience, the NIDA texts ultimately retreat to the neo-liberal project of CBT as the 'most effective treatment for methamphetamine addiction'.

Conclusion

Our focus in this chapter has been the collateral realities through which amphetamine dependence and methamphetamine addiction are constituted in two sets of documents: a series of influential research publications from the 1990s and two reports published by a key research agency in the 2000s. How do the themes we have explored in our analysis remake addiction? First, fear about methamphetamine use appears to be expanding the category of addiction. In the Australian texts, we see dependence being extended to those who do not fit the classic pattern of daily use but who use in an episodic or binge pattern. Yet even as this expansion is being enacted and stabilised, its central assumption – that compulsion is the key to understanding amphetamine dependence – becomes much less certain: in fact, Topp and Mattick call for further research on the:

> symptoms of a compulsion to use and salience of drug use in the user's life ... in order to assess the level of dependence of these individuals who, while less dependent than daily users, still manifest problematic patterns of use. (1997a, 160)

The NIDA texts also invoke a binge pattern of use as characteristic of methamphetamine addiction and, in the absence of evidence for physical withdrawal, offer an unprecedented and idiosyncratic definition of tolerance to explain compulsive use. In both sets of publications, addiction has been extended to a wider range of drug use practices and has come to be characterised by more complex distinctions. This move is far from politically neutral, as it allows greater numbers of people to be pathologised and thereby defined as in need of intervention.

Second, in both the Australian and American texts, dependence and addiction, as well as the harm arising from drug use, are enacted as anterior to, and independently of, attempts to identify and understand them. Epistemologically, the way to reveal these phenomena is through 'science' in the form of psychiatry, psychology, surveillance research and neuroscience. These ontological and epistemological assumptions are evident in the Australian texts' treatment of dependence on heroin and alcohol as an uncontroversial concept already settled by previous research. Later chapters will also explore the work done by new addiction debates to stabilise concepts otherwise regarded as controversial. The same ontological and epistemological assumptions are also evident in the 'fear' expressed in the NDARC technical report that existing research had failed to stabilise the 'nebulous' and 'contentious' amphetamine withdrawal syndrome. Indeed, the report's aim was to determine the very existence and dimensions of amphetamine dependence in order that drug policy and practice – both of which also work to produce stable objects (Bacchi 2009) – could begin developing effective responses. These ontological and epistemological assumptions are also evident in the NIDA texts' reliance on neuroscience's claim to unmediated access to an objective material world of primary qualities. In both cases, addiction needs to be defined as a stable object if it is to be addressed by policy and practice. But it is also stabilised as a particular type of object: one in which the 'social' is erased and with it the need to address complex social and political issues such as race, class, gender, inequality and marginalisation.

Our third concluding point concerns agency. In the Australian publications, a shift can be traced from classic models of heroin addiction to those relating to amphetamine dependence. Whereas in the former, agency was located primarily in the drug ('one shot and you're hooked'; 'it's so good, don't even try it once'), in the latter, the absence of physical withdrawal and patterns of non-daily use required that agency be relocated in the 'compulsive' drug-using subject. Agency is invoked quite differently in the NIDA texts on methamphetamine. Portrayed as potent, powerful and spreading across the nation, the drug remains, like heroin, the agent of addiction. Once consumed, methamphetamine's neurotoxic effects distort the natural functioning of the brain. Locating agency in these ways serves similar strategic and political ends to those noted above. It allocates responsibility for addiction to drugs or their consumers rather than understanding it as distributed across a range of complex phenomena, and allows for the development of policy and practice focused on supply and the treatment of pathological subjects.

Our final general point concerns pathology and politics. The extension of dependence and addiction to include non-daily, episodic forms of drug use is significant because it allows greater numbers of drug consumers, and a greater range of drug-use practices, to be pathologised. The SDS, a measurement tool widely used in research and clinical settings, is primarily suited to diagnosing flawed neo-liberal subjects, yet its ease of use in these settings allows ever greater numbers of 'dependent' drug consumers to be created, classified and managed. We can also see the influence of neo-liberal ideas and politics in the NIDA texts. Despite their championing of and reliance on neuroscience, they retreat to the neo-liberal project of CBT as the 'most effective treatment' for methamphetamine addiction.

The practices and collateral realities we have identified in these research texts are important because they have shaped the response to social and health issues relating to amphetamine and methamphetamine, allowed increasing numbers of drug consumers to be pathologised and enacted new realities of dependence and addiction. In the next chapter, we consider the extent to which the practices and collateral realities identified in psychological and neuroscientific research on amphetamine and methamphetamine inform the development of drug policy and its unique realities of addiction, and the collateral realities enacted by consumers of methamphetamine. How well do scientific realities hold together in the face of the many disparate and countervailing demands upon policy and methamphetamine consumers? How well do they serve the needs and limitations of policy and consumers?

3
Making Methamphetamine in Drug Policy and Consumer Accounts

In this chapter we build on the analysis of scientific research conducted in Chapter 2, focusing on the enactment of methamphetamine use and addiction in two further discursive contexts. First, drawing on Carol Bacchi's (2009, x) observation that policy does not simply 'address' issues and problems but actually 'shapes' them, we illuminate the collateral realities at work to stabilise methamphetamine use and addiction in drug policy, using Australia and the United States as case studies. The Australian and US policy documents we analyse were produced by a diverse range of stakeholders through complex processes of policy development and as such do not mirror each other in intention or in implicit and explicit approaches to methamphetamine use. All, however, are products of an imperative to 'address' such use. As such, they all face the same founding demand: they must establish and sustain their authority and legitimacy, even as, and especially because, the evidence they need to substantiate their necessary claim that methamphetamine use requires a strong policy response consistently proves elusive.

As we will argue, Australian policy echoes some of the collateral realities evident in the scientific literature: it enacts addiction as an unproblematic way of understanding methamphetamine use, collapses methamphetamine dependence and episodic use, equates methamphetamine use with harm and assumes the existence of effective treatment and other responses. We go on to argue that US policy enacts similarly questionable collateral realities: methamphetamine is a highly addictive and malevolent drug, and methamphetamine addiction is a brain disease. We show how the collateral realities of both Australian and US policy rely explicitly on the Australian and NIDA research we critiqued in the previous chapter, and consider the implications of these interlocking and mutually dependent collateral realities of addiction.

Our second area of investigation consists of accounts of methamphetamine use and addiction offered by those who consume the drug. We argue that consumer accounts both reproduce and challenge the collateral realities of methamphetamine use and addiction enacted in research (Chapter 2) and policy (this chapter). What are the similarities and differences in pathology, ontology, epistemology and agency in these accounts and what are their implications for contemporary understandings of addiction? In these accounts, methamphetamine use and addiction are co-produced in complex assemblages of biography, agency, subjectivity, normative expectations, material and discursive resources, pleasure and biomedical discourse. In analysing policy and consumer accounts, we consider how these collateral realities powerfully remake addiction in relation to methamphetamine.

Making methamphetamine in Australian drug policy

We begin by analysing the collateral realities at work to stabilise methamphetamine use and dependence[1] in three key Australian national and state policy documents dating from the late 2000s. The first document is a 20-page position paper on methamphetamines produced by the Australian National Council on Drugs (ANCD 2007), the Australian government's principal drug policy advisory body. The position paper's official status is conveyed by the ANCD name and Australian government coat of arms displayed on the first page. Following an Introduction, the document proceeds through several sections – covering, for example, patterns of use, medical and social problems, supply, prevention and treatment – before concluding with a list of 22 recommendations and 86 references. The text is broken up by highlighted and capitalised excerpts from the main text, and the insertion after each section of relevant recommendations from the final list appearing at the end of the paper. The second Australian policy document we analyse is the *National Amphetamine-Type Stimulant Strategy 2008–2011*, which includes extensive coverage of methamphetamine and carries the imprimatur of the Ministerial Council on Drug Strategy (MCDS) (2008).[2] The MCDS is the peak decision-making body on drug policy and practice and comprises the Australian, State and Territory Ministers of Health, Law Enforcement and Education. The report has just under 50 pages and consists of four sections – Introduction, Strategic Framework, Priority Areas and Where Next? – followed by 2 appendices and 34 references. The layout of the document is typical: an opening list of 29 acronyms, various levels of subheading, dot point and numbered lists, and tables summarising key information. The third document in which methamphetamine is a key focus emerges from state policy processes and was produced by the Victorian Department of Human Services (2008): the *Victorian Amphetamine-Type Stimulant (ATS) and Related Drugs Strategy 2009–2012*. The text's 41 pages consist of a Foreword from the Victorian Minister for Mental Health followed by an Introduction, coverage of five priority areas (prevention and early intervention, treatment, workforce development, justice and law enforcement, and new research and dissemination) and 22 references. This document also adopts the style for government reports: subheadings, dot point and numbered lists, and summary tables.

Before examining these policy documents in detail, some general points are worth making. The first is that, unlike almost all other published works, policy documents usually appear without named authorship. The opening pages of the documents nominate a body or committee from which the document has emerged, but do not identify the individuals who actively drafted the texts. This practice of leaving authorship unspecified has an important purpose in the processes of authorisation Bacchi (2009) identifies as part of policymaking. It aims to communicate neutrality, the notion that the contents of policy documents are not the product of individual interests or perspectives, of bias or politics, but of balanced, broad-based, disinterested bodies and committees acting responsibly and beyond the corrupting influence of the personal. The second is that these bodies and committees play an auspicing role in relation to the documents' contents, approach and conclusions. They generate authority by linking the contents to experts and other specialist stakeholders chosen as possessing a privileged relationship to the area of policy development. The effect of these strategies of anonymity and auspicing is that accountability for the texts is distributed and sequestered. Information about who has shaped the tone of the documents, the assumptions about the actions or effects of drugs from which they proceed, decisions about the status of data and evidence, and their approach to absences of data or evidence are all inaccessible except in very general terms. Likewise, the processes by which unexplained or undocumented steps in logic are introduced and permitted, that is, by which epistemological assumptions as to the relationship between particular concepts or actions are accepted by the authorship committees, remain opaque. Important processes by which the texts and their logics, and their relationship to other texts and to evidence, are submerged by this strategy. So too are specific avenues for communication about the documents, for questions about their aims, constitution and execution. In all these ways, the processes raise questions about neutrality, auspicing and accountability that are important to bear in mind when analysing the documents and considering how and to what extent they take possession of a privileged relationship to truth for professional readers and the general public.

In the following analysis we explore how these policy accounts stabilise their objects of concern: methamphetamine use and dependence. We argue that this stability is achieved and maintained through the following collateral realities:

- 'dependence' and 'addiction' are unproblematic ways of understanding methamphetamine;
- dependence and acute episodes of methamphetamine intoxication can be treated as a single category;
- methamphetamine use is linked to harm;
- knowledge is intrinsically cumulative; and
- effective policy and practice responses exist to address 'methamphetamine-related problems'.

The first collateral reality enacted in the policy documents is the installation of dependence and addiction as unproblematic ways of understanding methamphetamine use. As we will see in the sections below, all three documents take the existence of methamphetamine dependence for granted, omitting even the most rudimentary definitions of the term. In keeping with the aims of this book, we concentrate here on the invoking of addiction to methamphetamine. The Minister's Foreword to the *Victorian ATS Strategy* provides a vivid example of this, quoting an 'ice addict' and asserting the need for a 'pre-emptive strike on crystal meth' – a 'highly addictive drug'. The ANCD (2007, 1) position paper also produces methamphetamine as an 'addictive synthetic stimulant' and, later, as a 'highly addictive substance' (2007, 3). The validity of these formulations is, as we noted in Chapter 2, highly contestable. Indeed, the latter reference to methamphetamine as 'highly addictive' appears immediately after this sentence: 'Of the 1.5 million Australians who have tried methamphetamine, the majority has snorted or swallowed the drug on only a small number of occasions . . . and is unlikely to have experienced any significant problems from their methamphetamine use' (2007, 3). In what ways, then, is methamphetamine 'highly addictive' if most of those who take it are unlikely to have experienced significant problems? This glaring contradiction is never explained.

The highlighted text that appears in large capitals immediately to the left of this paragraph emphasises a very different aspect of the drug:

> ...METHAMPHETAMINE IS A HIGHLY ADDICTIVE SUBSTANCE, AND A PROPORTION OF PEOPLE WHO TRY THE DRUG MOVE ON TO TAKE METHAMPHETAMINE REGULARLY, OFTEN MAKING THE TRANSITION TO THE MORE EFFICIENT ROUTES OF SMOKING OR INJECTING THE DRUG.
>
> (ANCD 2007, 3)

Given the accompanying comments about the majority of those who consume the drug, the assertion that a 'proportion' move on to use methamphetamine 'regularly' is strikingly vague: is it 1%, 10%, 40%? To what group does the 'proportion' relate? The 1.5 million who have 'ever tried' methamphetamine, or the approximately 500,000 who have used it in the last 12 months? How is 'regularly' defined: temporally (daily, weekly, monthly) or contextually (each long weekend, each summer holiday, each dance party or rave)? The unspecified proportion that uses with undefined regularity 'often' makes the transition to smoking or injecting. How often is 'often'? How linear is this process? None of these important parameters of the nature or scale of the issues under discussion is clarified. Not only are glaring inconsistencies evident in the enactment of methamphetamine as 'highly addictive', but these are (rather obviously) managed by vague and inconclusive language.

A second collateral reality of methamphetamine in the three documents is the collapsing of methamphetamine dependence and episodic intoxication into a single category. The extension of dependence, and therefore of pathology, to include non-daily use of methamphetamine was also a feature of the Australian and NIDA publications we explored in the previous chapter. For example, the ANCD position paper argues for the need to adapt existing measures to methamphetamine as well as introducing some new measures. These new measures consist of three 'recent initiatives' responding to 'methamphetamine-specific issues'. The first initiative, 'guidelines on the frontline management of intoxicated individuals', presumably applies to all drugs, but here it appears to relate to methamphetamine psychosis, which is frequently highlighted as a key problem throughout the document (about which we say more below). Individuals experiencing methamphetamine intoxication are assumed to be paranoid, violent and psychotic and therefore pose greater problems in 'frontline' settings such as emergency departments and encounters with police. The second of the three initiatives comprises 'guidelines on the management of methamphetamine dependence'. The collapsing of dependence and episodic intoxication into a single category – or, at the very least, a blurring of the differences between the two – is achieved by the close textual positioning of the first initiative on the management of methamphetamine intoxication with the second initiative on the management of dependence.

A second example of the collapsing of dependence and episodic intoxication is found in the ANCD position paper in a section headed 'Preventing harms from methamphetamine use': 'Further preventative measures should target those groups most at risk of developing dependence or other adverse consequence[s] (e.g., psychosis) from their drug use' (ANCD 2007, 2). Here dependence is set against 'other adverse consequences' (although the two appear together), including psychosis. In the next section, however, psychosis is described as one of the problems 'related' to dependence. Thus in the first statement psychosis is a feature of non-dependent methamphetamine use, and in the second of dependent use. Claims that methamphetamine can produce psychosis irrespective of the patterns of its use enact the drug as different from amphetamine and as uniquely powerful.

The *National ATS Strategy* also collapses dependence and intoxication-related problems at several points. For example (MCDS 2008, 6):

> A large proportion of ATS dependent people will experience psychological problems including anxiety, depression and psychosis. Meth/amphetamine intoxication, and simultaneous use of other drugs, such as alcohol, and related agitation and aggression, impacts on frontline services (treatment centre, emergency departments and law enforcement) who report significant resource demands caused by amphetamine psychosis.

Here psychosis is one of the psychological problems experienced by a 'large proportion' of 'dependent people'. This implies that one needs to be dependent to experience psychosis. But then psychosis is also linked to episodic intoxication that impacts frontline services. Again, psychosis is mobilised to collapse dependence and intoxication into a single category.

The textual strategy in the policy documents through which psychosis is treated as an outcome common to both dependence and episodic intoxication reflects the various confusing ways in which psychosis is treated in the research literature. For example, both the ANCD position paper and the *National Strategy* extensively cite the research of

McKetin and colleagues. In one of these articles (McKetin, McLaren, Kelly, Lubman & Hides 2006), the authors argue that the prevalence of psychosis amongst 'regular' methamphetamine users is 11 times higher than amongst the general population in Australia, with 'regular' use being defined as 'at least monthly during the past year'. Here, psychosis appears to bridge, and strategically collapse, dependence and episodic use arising from recreational or binge patterns of methamphetamine consumption.

Another example of the way in which psychosis is mobilised to stabilise the reality of methamphetamine dependence or addiction, and to produce methamphetamine as different from amphetamine and as uniquely harmful, can be found in the Australian media campaign *Don't Let Ice Destroy You*, which was televised in 2007 and 2009 as part of the National Drugs Campaign. The footage depicted three images: a young man roughly pushing his mother; a woman aged in her 20s with her face covered in scars (apparently referencing the effects of skin picking due to 'formication', that is, the sensation of bugs crawling under the skin); and a shirtless young man in a hospital being restrained by police and security guards. The corresponding voice-over for this final scene declares solemnly: 'And then there's [*sic*] psychotic episodes. It's frightening that addiction can happen in such a short time' (accessed on 2 August 2013: www.couriermail.com.au/news/features/more-anti-drug-ads/story-fn2mcu0g-12257002944780). Here we see stark evidence of the collapsing of psychosis and addiction as a means of enacting the reality of methamphetamine addiction. If psychosis can arise following a single episode of use each month, in what way can the presence of psychosis be taken to constitute 'addiction'? And what does the evidence say, in any case, about the duration of methamphetamine use required to develop 'addiction'?

A third collateral reality at work in the policy documents is that methamphetamine use leads to harm. Consider this example from the ANCD position paper (2007, 1):

> The major public health consequences related to methamphetamine use occur disproportionately among people who are dependent on the drug. Harms associated with heavy methamphetamine use include psychotic symptoms (paranoia and hallucinations), crime (drug dealing, property crime), aggression or violent behaviour (particularly during drug-induced psychosis), deterioration in social functioning, and a range of physical health problems (stroke, cardiovascular pathology, dental problems).

This statement displays considerable slippage between causation, forms of use and types of harm. No references are provided to support the various claims made. 'Major public health consequences' are not defined but are 'related to methamphetamine use' rather than dependence. These consequences are worse for those who are 'dependent' (again not defined), but the specific harms listed are 'associated with heavy methamphetamine use', which is treated as being equivalent to dependent use. Of the harms, psychotic symptoms are again given prominence and, later in the list, we are told aggression or violence arises 'particularly' from 'drug-induced psychosis'. The list also includes crime, and specifically drug dealing, but of course the crime of drug dealing must, by definition, be associated with all prohibited drugs. So, we have three different categories of use – 'use', 'dependent' and 'heavy' – and several forms of relationship – 'consequences', 'related to', 'associated with' and 'drug-induced'.

The ANCD position paper, although also enacting this collateral reality of methamphetamine's harmfulness, provides a second example of the loose treatment of evidence, this time in relation to causation (2007, 1):

> Fatalities from methamphetamine use are not common, and less likely than for heroin use, for example (5). However, methamphetamine does increase the risk of stroke and cardiac failure (6, 7), and a notable number of methamphetamine-related deaths have been documented in parts of the US where the drug's use is common. In Australia there are currently around 50 deaths a year that are attributed directly to the use of psychostimulant drugs, including methamphetamine (8).

First, the choice of language on frequency is worth examining closely. Rather than 'rare', deaths from methamphetamine use are 'not common'. What constitutes 'common' and, by implication, 'not common' is not quantified and the single cited reference (5 in the above quotation) is a study conducted amongst heroin and amphetamine (rather than methamphetamine) users in Perth, Western Australia, between 1985 and 1998 (Bartu et al. 2004). It is hard to escape the conclusion here that the more appropriate word, 'rare', is avoided because it is not sufficiently alarming. In the United States, a 'notable number' of 'methamphetamine-related' deaths have occurred but no specific number or reference is provided – so the number could just as easily be 'notably' low. In Australia, 'around 50 deaths a year...are attributed directly to the use of psychostimulant drugs'. No details are provided on several key issues in relation to this statement: the criteria for attributing deaths to psychostimulant drugs, who makes this assessment or the proportion of 'psychostimulant' deaths attributed 'directly' to methamphetamine – is it 5%, 30%, 75%? – as opposed to the other drugs included in the category of psychostimulant (such as cocaine). The cited reference (8 in the above quotation) is an unrefereed technical report that focuses on 'cocaine and amphetamine [rather than methamphetamine] mentions in accidental drug-induced deaths in Australia' between 1997 and 2003 (Degenhardt et al. 2003).

A third example of the loose use of evidence in relation to methamphetamine and harm in the ANCD position paper can be found in the following claim: 'The harms caused by chronic methamphetamine use upon [*sic*] the families and friends of the user also need to be recognised and addressed' (ANCD 2007, 9). What does this sentence mean? It does not refer to 'dependent' drug use, although chronicity in the form of daily use is a hallmark of original definitions of dependence. And whereas in earlier framings, methamphetamine is 'related to' or 'associated with' specific forms of harm, here it 'causes' harm 'upon' others. Despite this more strongly expressed association, the evidence presented for the claim in the next sentence – 'anecdotal reports of disturbance and distress' – is less than conclusive.

Unlike the ANCD position paper, the *National Strategy* uses the generic term 'amphetamine-type stimulants' or 'ATS', defining the 'main ATS used' in Australia as methamphetamine and ecstasy. It also takes a much more cautious approach to the question of evidence than the ANCD document. For example, both the website and the *National Strategy* document note (Department of Health and Ageing n.d., 6):

> There are particular challenges associated with treating ATS dependence and related problems but the evidence-base to support the development and implementation of specific interventions has been limited, especially when compared to other drugs such as tobacco, alcohol or heroin.

The expression 'evidence-base' invites scrutiny in that it carries a range of assumptions. Some of these are straightforwardly positivist – for example, in their faith in objectivity and the possibility of value-free knowledge. Other assumptions are specific to the context: how much evidence constitutes a 'base' in this field? Indeed, what is a base in this field? What does the idea of a base assume about the production of drug policy? If we look elsewhere on the website, we find clues as to the answers to these questions. For example, the introduction states:

> A large proportion of people affected by ATS use (i.e. those who are not severely dependent and who are not experiencing severe problems) are suitable for opportunistic brief interventions and there is an evidence base to guide such interventions.

What does this particular evidence base comprise? The statement itself is not supported by a citation, and the reference list that appears below the text contains only one citation on the topic, an unrefereed research monograph (Baker, Lee & Jenner 2004). As we noted in Chapter 2, this research monograph occupies a prominent position in all three policy documents and relies explicitly on the NDARC research. As one of the monograph editors states: 'Although psychostimulant use tends to be characterised by intermittent rather than daily use, a clear dependence syndrome has been described (e.g. Topp & Mattick, 1997b)' (Lee 2004, 56). The body of the *National Strategy* document does not provide any further support for the claim that an evidence base exists; indeed, very few references appear in the document as a whole (the entire bibliography comprises only 34 sources).

Further to the *National Strategy's* approach to evidence, the Executive Summary concedes: 'Some evidence about the adverse consequences of ATS use has only recently emerged, and there are still gaps in knowledge' (2008, 11). This statement is valuable in its gesture towards the unknowns of ATS such as methamphetamine. Yet our enquiry into the meaning of evidence in this area of policy leads us to query a key term here. What, we ask, is a 'gap'? This is a potent image that communicates much about the nature of reality and of knowledge about it. Is the field described here sufficiently populated with widely agreed-upon knowledge that only gaps remain? We would argue that this expression significantly under-represents the extent of what is not known about ATS, and in the process produces a collateral reality in which knowledge is treated as intrinsically cumulative. In Bacchi's (2009) terms, this language presupposes a broad extant base of evidence, leaves unproblematised issues to do with the constraints on the production of evidence – such as the limits of research funding and the role of public opinion in shaping research priorities – and produces knowledge about ATS as almost complete, rather than rudimentary, patchy and therefore unreliable. In a context where research is relatively thin, and individual studies are used to justify broad statements about the nature of drug problems and significant policy decisions, this theory of reality is of great utility. Thin research, in this logic, is not overturned by new findings (rendering decisions based on it invalid); new findings simply add to those already accepted. They confirm that which has already been used, despite its contingency, to shape policy.

The final collateral reality at work in the Australian drug policy documents is that there exist effective treatment responses to 'methamphetamine-related problems'. Consider the following example from the *National Strategy*:

> While there is limited evidence about treatment strategies that are specific to ATS dependence, many approaches have been effectively used with other drugs and *it is anticipated that these can be adapted and transferred* to prevent and reduce ATS problems [emphasis added]. (2008, 25)

Thus the *National Strategy* takes a somewhat confused approach to the issue of treatment for dependence. It is cautious in noting the limited evidence in relation to the treatment of ATS dependence but also optimistically claims that there are effective treatments for other drugs and that these are relevant to ATS. As Ritter and Lintzeris (2004) have cautioned, however, only 30% of those individuals undergoing drug addiction treatment are likely to reduce the harm associated with their use. The document then strikes a rather optimistic note when it 'anticipates' that such treatments can be successfully adapted and transferred to ATS, even as methamphetamine is consistently treated as a unique problem (as we saw, for example, in relation to psychosis).

If the *National Strategy* is by turns cautious, optimistic and hopeful on the issue of treatment, the same cannot be said for the ANCD position paper. The section on 'Treatment for methamphetamine dependence' opens with rather more unequivocal statements (the first two sentences also appear in bold capitals in an accompanying text box):

> Improving treatment coverage for methamphetamine dependence should be a first priority. Reducing the number of people who are dependent on the drug will reduce the incidence of psychosis, crime, and violent behaviour associated with methamphetamine use. We have effective treatments for methamphetamine dependence,

> which have been developed and evaluated in Australia, and these should be implemented broadly and in a way that is readily accessible to methamphetamine users.
>
> (ANCD 2007, 2)

What are these effective treatments? The earlier reference to treatment states that these include 'psychosocial treatments', but these are not spelt out. They are not described and no references are cited for their evaluation as effective. Later, the paper states somewhat contradictorily that '[c]urrently few treatment approaches for methamphetamine dependence have been comprehensively evaluated' (ANCD 2007, 10). In policy terms, constructing methamphetamine use and dependence as a problem requires that solutions be offered. But why advocate improved treatment coverage in the absence of conclusive evidence for its success?

If we investigate further the evidence offered in the ANCD position paper for its collateral reality of effective responses for methamphetamine dependence, we find that 'psychosocial treatments' refer mainly to cognitive behavioural therapy (CBT), and the cited reference for CBT's effectiveness is a chapter in the 2004 monograph cited earlier (Baker, Gowing et al. 2004). Yet if we return to the careful conclusions of the authors of this chapter (2004, 82), we find:

> The literature on amphetamine treatments is *limited in both quantity and quality*. The literature is particularly *hindered by a paucity of well-conducted studies among primary amphetamine users, especially outcome studies*. The *available evidence suggests that* cognitive behavioural approaches, such as relapse prevention, and behavioural approaches, such as contingency management, are the most effective treatments for amphetamine users *to date*. The effectiveness of other types of intervention *is not well supported*. Until more research is undertaken comparing different treatment modalities in Australian settings, CBT, coupled with motivational approaches, *appears to represent current best practice* [emphasis added].

Hardly a ringing endorsement of the evidence base.

The *Victorian ATS Strategy* is similarly bullish in its advocacy of treatment:

> A stepped care approach has been identified as an appropriate response for ATS users. This approach first offers the least

> intensive intervention that is likely to be effective and then involves more intensive interventions, if required (Baker et al. 2005). (2008, 20)
>
> There is a substantial body of evidence that demonstrates the efficacy of CBT, motivational interviewing and other psychosocial therapies with ATS users (Topp 2006). (2008, 20)

The solitary reference offered in support of a stepped care approach – Baker et al. (2005) – is a single randomised-controlled trial undertaken in Newcastle in which the success of the intervention was evaluated at six-month follow-up. The reference for the 'substantial body of evidence' – Topp (2006) – is an unrefereed article in an alcohol and other drug sector publication which consists of interviews with key treatment figures in the field and several references to the Baker et al. (2005) article.

Later in the *Victorian Strategy* document, in the section on 'Psychosocial treatment', we learn:

> Current evidence indicates that CBT is the most effective treatment for methamphetamine users. The approach to working with regular methamphetamine users, including hazardous, harmful or dependent users, may include a combination of interventions, such as motivational interviewing techniques, used in conjunction with behavioural interventions.
>
> A stepped care approach is considered most effective in better matching treatment to a client's needs and readiness to change, whereby each incremental step is made available on the basis of the client's response to the previous one.
>
> The *Methamphetamine dependence and treatment clinical guidelines*...suggest using primarily psychosocial interventions such as CBT and motivational interviewing to manage withdrawal from methamphetamine. (2008, 23)

In the *Victorian Strategy* paper the provisional nature and cautious recommendations of Baker et al. (2004, 2005) are, to use Law's phrase, 'washed away', as they were in the ANCD document. Why draw attention to expressions of increasing certainty regarding the effectiveness of treatment across a chain of several linked documents? The process has, we argue, specific political effects. The collateral reality of treatment effectiveness increasingly established in the various documents remakes service provision in very specific ways – for example, in the establishment of a trial of two 'specialist methamphetamine health centres' in Melbourne and in the creation of specific clinical guidelines for the management of 'methamphetamine-dependent clients' (2008, 23). All these in turn re-enact the problem of methamphetamine and ATS.

A clear example of this remaking of service provision can be found in the Strategy's 'key actions', which embrace brief interventions and CBT despite the relative paucity of evidence:

> 2.2 Through workforce development strengthen the capacity of the [alcohol and other drug] sector to provide psychological interventions, particularly brief interventions, to ATS and related drug users.
>
> 2.3 Promote compliance with the existing *Methamphetamine dependence and treatment clinical guidelines* (see Box 2) within the [alcohol and other drug] sector.

Box 2 collapses dependence and episodic or 'acute' methamphetamine use (as well as unqualified 'use') under clinical guidelines for 'methamphetamine dependence and treatment':

- tools to manage acute presentations – toxicity, aggressive behaviour and psychotic symptoms;
- interventions for use and dependence – assessment, managing withdrawal, reducing harms, brief interventions and CBT.

Here we see distinct political effects of the enactment of certainty about the effectiveness of treatment, in that it shapes the definition, classification and management of 'dependent' subjects.

In summary, the three Australian policy documents we have analysed are products of an imperative to 'address' methamphetamine use and dependence as issues of sufficient severity to warrant extended policy attention. They must establish and sustain their authority and legitimacy, even as, and especially because, the evidence they need to substantiate the claims that methamphetamine deserves such attention, and that effective responses are available, consistently proves elusive. This process of authorisation and legitimisation is maintained in several ways. First, dependence and addiction are enacted as ontologically unproblematic ways of understanding methamphetamine. However, the documents fail to clarify, or contain glaring contradictions in, the evidence cited for the nature or scale of dependence and addiction. Second, as we saw with the Australian and NIDA research publications in Chapter 2, the three policy documents collapse methamphetamine dependence and episodic intoxication. Psychosis plays a crucial role in stabilising the object of methamphetamine addiction, and of methamphetamine as different from amphetamine and other drugs, and as uniquely harmful, in relation to both 'dependent' and 'regular' use. The third collateral reality helping to stabilise methamphetamine use and addiction is epistemological. Methamphetamine use and addiction are frequently linked to various forms of harm, but the evidence for this relationship is absent, inadequate or contradictory, key terms and forms of drug use are left undefined, and the relationship between harm and the drug is described in diverse ways: as consequential, 'related to', 'associated with', 'caused by' and 'induced by'. That knowledge is intrinsically cumulative is a fourth collateral reality used to stabilise this object. It assumes that objective, value-free knowledge is possible, that even scant knowledge about a topic can be described as an 'evidence base', and that only 'gaps' in our knowledge of methamphetamine remain (an alternative metaphor for the state of the evidence could, for example, be 'islands' of knowledge in a vast 'sea' of unknowns). Finally, stabilising methamphetamine use and dependence in Australian policy involves claims about the existence of effective responses to 'methamphetamine-related problems'. In policy terms, constructing methamphetamine use and dependence as a unique problem requires that solutions be available. But again, when scrutinised carefully, the cited 'substantial' evidence base turns out to be absent, limited or provisional even as it remakes service provision and the problem of methamphetamine use in specific ways.

To what extent do the collateral realities we have identified in Australian policy emerge beyond this context? How well is the object of methamphetamine addiction holding together internationally? In the next section, we consider the stabilisation and collateral realities of methamphetamine use and addiction in policy documents published by the United States Office of National Drug Control Policy (ONDCP), which is part of the Executive Office of the US President. Like their Australian counterparts, the ONDCP documents must authorise and legitimise the claim that methamphetamine deserves extended policy consideration, but the collateral realities they enact along the way, influenced as they are by the NIDA research analysed in Chapter 2, differ in some important ways from those found in the Australian texts.

Making methamphetamine in US national drug policy

According to its website (accessed on 2 August 2013: www.whitehouse.gov/ondcp/about), the ONDCP

> advises the President on drug-control issues, coordinates drug-control activities and related funding across the Federal government, and produces the annual National Drug Control Strategy, which outlines Administration efforts to reduce illicit drug use, manufacturing and trafficking, drug-related crime and violence, and drug-related health consequences.[3]

The ONDCP documents we analyse here deal with drug use and addiction in general as well as methamphetamine in particular. We take this approach because the methamphetamine-specific material draws on, and elaborates, the themes evident in the general policy documents. We argue that the discursive practices at work in these documents constitute the following collateral realities:

- addiction is a brain disease being progressively revealed by advances in neuroscience;
- methamphetamine is highly addictive; and
- methamphetamine is a malevolent agent.

We begin our analysis by examining how the 2012 National Drug Control Strategy and other ONDCP documents treat addiction. First, unlike Australian policy which, as we have noted, largely overlooks the emerging neuroscience of addiction, these documents echo strongly the unquestioning faith in (neuro)science displayed in the NIDA documents we analysed in Chapter 2. This debt to NIDA orthodoxy is made explicit in several places. For example, the ONDCP home page features a video clip of NIDA Director and neuroscientist Nora Volkow discussing the neuroscience of addiction (accessed on 28 August 2013), and we learn from the 'fact sheet' summarising the key elements of the Strategy:

> Decades of scientific study show that drug addiction is not a moral failing on the part of the individual – but a *disease of the brain* that can be prevented and treated [emphasis added].
>
> (Accessed on 2 August 2013: www.whitehouse.gov/ondcp/ondcp-fact-sheets/our-strategy)

Clicking on the *underlined* text in the above quotation redirects the reader to the NIDA website and a page headed 'DrugFacts: Understanding Drug Abuse and Addiction'. In a sidebar on the right-hand side of the web page, there is an image of the front cover of *Drugs, Brains, and Behavior: The Science of Addiction* (NIDA 2010b). As we noted in Chapter 2, this publication sets out NIDA's position on drug use and addiction, which emphasises the collateral reality of neuroscience as an explanatory framework and ignores any consideration of the social. On this web page, addiction is defined as a 'chronic, *often* [emphasis added] relapsing brain disease that causes compulsive drug seeking and use, despite harmful consequences to the addicted individual and to those around him or her'. This is an interesting and unusual use of 'often'. What purpose could it serve? It might be intended to minimise fatalism among members of the public visiting the page by suggesting that the chronic disease of addiction does not *always* lead to relapse. But it also raises the question of whether addiction exists in the absence of relapse. If a person taking drugs is asked to stop, and this cessation is achieved without relapse, is this addiction?

Further examples of the Strategy's debt to NIDA's advocacy of neuroscience appear in other parts of the ONDCP website. For instance:

> [The Strategy] rejects the false choice between an enforcement-centric 'war on drugs' and the extreme notion of drug legalization. Science has shown that *drug addiction is not a moral failing but rather a disease of the brain* that can be prevented and treated [emphasis added].
>
> (Accessed on 2 August 2013: www.whitehouse.gov/ondcp/2012-national-drug-control-strategy)

Similarly, the press release accompanying the Strategy quotes Gil Kerlikowske, Director of National Drug Control Policy:

> The policy alternatives contained in our new *Strategy* support mainstream reforms based on *the proven facts that drug addiction is a disease of the brain* that can be prevented and treated and that we cannot simply arrest our way out of the drug problem [emphasis added].
>
> (Accessed on 11 December 2012: www.whitehouse.gov/ondcp/ondcp/news-releases-remarks/obama-administration-releases-21st-century-drug-policy-strategy)

In these excerpts, an apparently neutral and monolithic '[neuro]science' provides an enlightened alternative – in the form of 'proven facts' – to the 'false choice' between 'war' and 'legalization'.

In the same press release, Stuart Gitlow, Acting President of the American Society of Addiction Medicine, provides further support for the enlightening potential and practical application of a neuroscientific understanding of addiction when he states:

> Advances in neurosciences over the past decades have provided us with invaluable insight into our Nation's drug problem... We are pleased the Obama administration's approach to drug control treats *drug addiction as a chronic disease of the brain rather than a behavioral problem on the part of the individual.* We commend their efforts to put in place evidence-based public health solutions that will help bring those suffering from substance abuse disorders get [*sic*] the treatment they need to recover and lead healthy lives free from addiction [emphasis added].

In this excerpt, we see (i) further enactment of the collateral reality of addiction as a brain disease and (ii) an additional collateral reality under enactment: that those with 'substance use disorders' should receive appropriate treatment. A further collateral reality enacted in the latter collateral reality is that effective treatment options exist. As we noted in Chapter 2, the evidence for the effectiveness of available drug treatments is modest at best, and brain science, the centrepiece of NIDA's approach to drug use and addiction, has so far failed to deliver new treatments.

In view of the numerous enactments of addiction as a brain disease on the ONDCP website, and the links to NIDA's website, it is surprising to find that there are no references to the terms 'neuroscience' or 'brain' in the 69-page written version of the Strategy, and a mere 20 references to addiction, which are mainly descriptive (for example, 'addiction services' or 'addiction treatment'). Addiction is defined once and then only briefly (ONDCP 2012, 23):

> By *recognizing drug addiction as a chronic and progressive disease* and working to prevent and treat the *underlying substance use disorder,* drug related crime and recidivism can be reduced [emphasis added].

As in the excerpts cited above, addiction is produced in this statement as a disorder underlying – that is, as ontologically prior to – its manifestation in social issues such as crime.[4] Here, addiction is cast not as a brain disease but as a 'chronic and progressive disease' – an underlying substance use disorder. The absence of neuroscience here is puzzling, but one reason for this silence could be that neuroscience presently offers few concrete policy directions.

If we consider the methamphetamine-specific material on the ONDCP website, the first thing to note is its relative paucity. This seems odd given the unequivocal view of US Attorney General Alberto Gonzales (cited in Chapter 2) that 'in terms of damage to children and to our society, meth is now the most dangerous drug in America', and also given NIDA's portrayal of methamphetamine's addictiveness and potency. However, where methamphetamine does appear, it does so in stark terms that reiterate its seriousness, addicting qualities and worthiness as a legitimate focus of policy. Here we see a second collateral reality helping to stabilise methamphetamine addiction: that the drug is highly addictive. Consider the following extract from the ONDCP web page containing introductory material on methamphetamine (accessed on 2 August 2013: www.whitehouse.gov/ondcp/meth-intro):

> Meth is an addictive stimulant drug that strongly activates certain systems in the brain and has a high potential for abuse.

Furthermore:

> Methamphetamine comes in more than one form – it can be smoked, snorted, injected, or orally ingested, though smoking has become more common recently. Smoking leads to very fast intake into the brain, which multiplies the user's potential for addiction and health implications.

The links at the bottom of the web page reinforce the emphasis on methamphetamine's impact on the brain. These links take the reader to the NIDA publications on methamphetamine we analysed in Chapter 2, with two of the links leading directly to the same NIDA report (NIDA 2006a).

What should we make of the inconsistent language used in these ONDCP statements? In the first, addictiveness is a defining feature of 'meth', but the language used is vague: it 'strongly activates certain systems in the brain' and has 'high potential for abuse'. In the second quotation, methamphetamine 'multiplies the user's potential' for addiction – multiplies by what factor? Two, ten, 50? Is this an attempt to sound 'scientific' rather than using everyday language such as 'increases'? If methamphetamine only multiplies the 'potential' for addiction, does it make sense to define it as 'addictive'? How, in short, should methamphetamine be understood?

Within the text on the 'meth-intro' page is a link to another section of the ONDCP website containing information on the National Youth Anti-Drug Media Campaign. Within this section is a subsection entitled 'Get the Drug Facts', which covers a wide range of licit and illicit drugs. The information the 'Meth' link provides reiterates the evocative language of the introductory material discussed above, but in this text the language is much more consistently pathologising. The first line states that the drug is '[h]ighly addictive and toxic [i.e. poisonous] to the brain' and 'will give you a high that can damage your body and brain for life'. There is little or no equivocation here. Further down the page, we are told (again):

> Meth, or methamphetamine, is a powerfully addictive stimulant that is both long-lasting and toxic to the brain. Its chemistry is similar to speed (amphetamine), but meth has far more dangerous effects on the body's central nervous system.
>
> (Accessed on 2 August 2013: www.abovetheinfluence.com/facts/drugsmeth)

This time 'addictive' or even 'highly addictive' are insufficient descriptors, with meth being redefined as 'powerfully addictive'. Despite its chemical resemblance to amphetamine, its effects are 'far more dangerous', but readers are not told why or in what ways. Could it be because youth – understood as innocent, passive and susceptible to peer pressure, yet also the focus of repeated waves of concern – is the subject of these pages?

In these various ONDCP extracts, the potential for addiction is explained entirely through the route of ingestion, pharmacology and neuroscience. As we noted in Chapter 2, qualitative research on the social contexts and cultural meanings of methamphetamine use is entirely absent from this discussion. As a result, the 'social' is erased from its causal accounts and, in turn, the need to address broad social issues, such as race, class, gender, inequality and marginalisation, that necessarily form part of the assemblage of drug use. Instead, several narrowing collateral realities are enacted: the brain as an apolitical, neutral space or object; the drug as the sole active agent; and the 'toxic' effects of drugs as unequivocal and permanent.

In positioning methamphetamine as highly addictive, the ONDCP texts also enact another collateral reality: methamphetamine is a malevolent agent. Take, for example, the following extract:

> The production and use of methamphetamine is a serious threat to the health and safety of our communities... Most of the methamphetamine abused in this country comes from foreign or domestic superlabs, although it can also be made in small, illegal laboratories, where its production endangers the people in the labs, neighbors, and the environment.
>
> (Accessed on 2 August 2013: www.whitehouse.gov/ondcp/meth-intro)

What exactly is a 'superlab' and how does it differ from an ordinary laboratory? Why the reference to 'foreign' labs? That the labs are either domestic or foreign is self-evident, but the sentence allows the introduction of the idea that the source of trouble could be foreigners. The tone here is implicitly xenophobic – addiction arises in part from the actions of unscrupulous outsiders endangering neutral, innocent (American) brains. Even methamphetamine's very production 'endangers' humans (and does not distinguish between 'criminals' engaged in methamphetamine manufacture and 'innocent' neighbours) and the environment.

In another section of the website, in which youth are singled out as a specific risk category, methamphetamine's malevolent agency is again highlighted:

> Since 2007, the National Youth Anti-Drug Media Campaign has supported a national Anti-Meth Campaign through TV, radio, print, and online anti-meth advertising in *areas of the country hardest hit by meth* [emphasis added].
>
> (Accessed on 2 August 2013: www.whitehouse.gov/ondcp/meth-intro)

Here methamphetamine is likened to a natural disaster such as a hurricane or flood – an act of God beyond human understanding and control that can wreak terrible destruction. In a country regularly exposed to death and destruction in relation to natural disasters, such imagery is extremely evocative. Indeed, 2005's Hurricane Katrina comes to mind here: it too was a disaster in which the mobilisation of the 'natural' was seen by some to cover over the political basis for the harms experienced (Sharkey 2007).

The 'Drug Facts' section we discussed above also positions methamphetamine as a malevolent agent. Consider the following descriptions of its effects and capacities:

> Meth *works by severely changing* the way the brain functions. First, it *increases* the release of the brain chemical dopamine. At the same time, it *blocks* the brain from absorbing the dopamine released [emphasis added].
>
> Because it's such a *highly addictive drug,* using meth a few times can lead to getting hooked – and the long-term effects of this drug are *ugly and scary. It can make you* lose weight, lose your teeth and develop scabs and open sores on your skin and face. Chronic meth abusers can become anxious and violent. Meth users often display a range of psychotic behaviors, including paranoia, hallucinations and delusions. One of the most common meth delusions is the feeling of insects crawling under the skin [emphasis added].
>
> *Powerfully addictive and powerfully damaging* to your body and brain – you might ask yourself if meth is really worth the risk. If you get hooked, *paranoia, skin scabs and a toothless 'meth mouth'* might be the best you'll get out of the deal. But *long-term brain damage and death* are the risks you also take [emphasis added].
>
> (Accessed on 2 August 2013: www.abovetheinfluence.com/facts/drugsmeth)

Such strong language and images are quite shocking to the contemporary eye, bringing to mind as they do the widely lampooned 'Reefer Madness' messages of the past. Methamphetamine is nevertheless produced as a powerful, pathological, destructive force with ugly and scary effects. Once inside the human body, it changes brains by increasing dopamine production and blocking its re-uptake; it hooks the consumer after only a few instances of use; it makes one lose weight and teeth, and become violent, psychotic and delusional; and its long-term legacy is brain damage and death. As with the authorising strategies mobilised in Australian policy documents, nowhere in these pages do we find definitions or supporting statistics on the prevalence of these extreme forms of harm. Instead they function via a kind of self-evident truth – the collateral reality of malevolence – about methamphetamine that operates above and beyond the need for evidence.

In summary, the ONDCP documents, like their Australian counterparts, work to authorise and legitimise the claim that methamphetamine use and addiction are serious, indeed alarming, issues that deserve extended policy consideration even as they are accompanied by little supporting research and able to offer only limited policy responses. However, unlike the Australian documents, in which several complex discursive dynamics are evident, the US policy documents make a narrower range of claims, strident and unequivocal, that admit little ambiguity. First, the collateral reality of drug addiction is constituted – through an epistemology that privileges the proven facts of a politically neutral and monolithic neuroscience – as a brain disorder 'underlying' (that is, as ontologically prior to) its manifestation in social issues. Second, the documents enact the collateral reality of methamphetamine as highly addictive and thus a legitimate focus of policy, with its potential for addiction explicable through the route of ingestion, pharmacology and neuroscience. The 'social' is erased and with it the need to address social issues such as race, class, gender, inequality and marginalisation. The final collateral reality helping to stabilise methamphetamine use and addiction in the ONDCP documents is the positioning of methamphetamine as a malevolent agent, comparable to a natural disaster, endangering human health and the environment, and leaving a terrible legacy of pathological subjects who have died or who continue to suffer from brain damage. What other ways of thinking about methamphetamine use and addiction do these strategies close off? What habits of thought do they rely upon and reproduce? Understanding addiction exclusively as a brain disease or the inevitable outcome of malign chemistry, or drugs as akin to natural disasters or malevolent agents, renders unnecessary attempts to understand addiction as arising from complex assemblages. While neuroscientific accounts might appear at first sight to constitute a 'new' way of understanding human experience, they are instead, as many have noted (Latour 2004; Rose 2006), an extension of long-standing biologically determinist ways of enacting the world. Understanding addiction this way allows policy to ignore the diverse, complex and potentially thorny social issues that shape drug problems.

In the next section, we examine the experiences and perspectives of methamphetamine consumers. What aspects of drug use do these accounts enact? What alternative collateral realities of drug use do they make available for research, policy and practice? And to what extent are the collateral realities enacted in psychological and neuroscientific research (Chapter 2) and policy (this chapter) also observable in the accounts of those who consume methamphetamine? What are the similarities and differences in ontology, epistemology, pathology and agency in these consumer accounts?

Consuming methamphetamine

In Chapter 2 and in the previous sections of this chapter, we argued that drug research and policy produces addiction as ontologically anterior to the social circumstances in which it unfolds; adopts an epistemology that positions addiction as discoverable through attention to psychology, pharmacology or neuroscience; redefines addiction to methamphetamine as including episodic patterns of use in addition to daily, chronic use, and thereby extends the reach of pathology; produces methamphetamine as highly addictive; and locates agency in either the 'compulsive' (that is, pathological) desires of consumers or their brains, or in the (malevolent) drug itself. The consumer interview material we turn to now both reproduces and challenges the ways in which methamphetamine and addiction are produced in research and policy practices.

Drawn from the ethnographic component of an ethno-epidemiological study investigating methamphetamine use and service provision in Melbourne, Australia, the consumer accounts of methamphetamine use we analyse here were collected in 31 semi-structured, in-depth interviews and participant observation across a range of sites (for details of data collection and analysis, see the Appendix). Of the many themes discussed in the interviews (drug use history, current methamphetamine use, experiences of service provision and so on), we focus on three collateral realities they enacted: methamphetamine use and addiction are complex phenomena, methamphetamine use is a 'habit' and methamphetamine use affects the brain. These speak most clearly to our identified concerns in this book.

When asked about the 'kinds of problems', if any, that they had experienced with methamphetamine, most interviewees used the term 'addiction'. The meanings attached to this word were many and varied, and the complex collateral realities of addiction they enacted both echoed and differed from those of research and policy. First, consumers differentiated sharply between 'physical' and psychological addiction, linking the former to opiates and the latter to methamphetamine. Mike (a 25-year-old man) commented:

> You know I kind of laugh when people say they're addicted to it [methamphetamine] because I just think of how addictive the morphine was and it's like 'well you think you've got an addiction, go on morphine and you'll find out [about] addiction'... you'll be in pain every day and you won't be able to eat until you have your hit

> and it's like you won't be able to do anything, you know, you'll be just destroyed. You think you've got no energy now, go on heroin and [...you'll] know pain then.

Mike went on to claim:

> I can't say I'm addicted to it [methamphetamine] because I know scientifically there's no such thing as being addicted to an amphetamine of any sort because it's all in the head, that's the addiction. It's not really addiction. What scientifically doctors call addiction is hanging for it body-wise. You get sick for it like heroin. That's addiction. That's how we define addiction scientifically.

Mike's views suggest a good deal of exposure to the collateral realities of scientific and treatment discourse on addiction, and a strong sense of clarity about the meaning of addiction. In this respect he differs sharply from the women we discuss in Chapter 7, who, in talking about overeating and obesity, rarely expressed certainty about addiction to anything. Mike's comments also position him as a member of a community of knowledge that includes not only scientists but also consumers.

Like Mike, Tanya (47 years old) distinguished between physical and psychological addiction:

> [I had a] psychological addiction [to methamphetamine] because you can't get addicted physically to it. People's aches and pains that they think are withdrawal symptoms... but I try to explain to them that our bodies are designed to rest up when you sleep and because we're using speed our muscles [...] aren't getting that rest, so that's where the aches and pains come from.

Tanya's comments also suggest exposure to some of the collateral realities of science and treatment (for example, that addiction is a real, anterior state directly related to certain substances) but not others (for example, accounts of methamphetamine as a drug of 'addiction'). Unlike Mike, her community of knowledge extends only to fellow consumers.

Similarly, Jim (41 years old) questioned the idea of physical addiction to methamphetamine:

> I don't believe that ice or speed is addictive. I think it's all [a] state of mind, it's not a physical [thing], you know. Like, you spend years

> on smack and you notice when you don't have it, you know, whereas [with] speed it's, you know like, take a few valium and just have a good sleep and just chill. Have something to eat...I just call them [people who claim to be addicted to methamphetamine] full of shit. It's not an addictive drug.

Like Tanya and Mike, Jim's comments suggest considerable exposure to prevailing collateral realities of methamphetamine addiction and, like Tanya, he defines his community of knowledge as limited to fellow consumers.

Although our interviewees emphasised a psychological component to methamphetamine addiction, closer inspection suggests a complex field of ideas around the psyche or mind. When asked to elaborate on what they meant by 'psychological' addiction, several seemed ambivalent about whether they were in fact 'addicted' in any way. Take Phil (a 26-year-old man), for example:

> Well supposedly you can [get addicted to methamphetamine] but I don't really think you can...Maybe mentally addicted to it but, like, heroin is a physical addiction where if you don't have it, you're curling up in a ball crying your eyes out because you're so sick. Speed and that, see I've binged on it and, you know, sort of every day for months, and I've never sort of felt any addiction to it.

When asked to elaborate on what they meant by 'addiction' to methamphetamine, other interviewees described feeling 'agitated', having 'low energy', feeling a 'little bit lethargic' or 'coming down' following methamphetamine use. For them, the remedy for methamphetamine's psychological addiction was relatively straightforward:

> You have a good sleep and you're fine. (Tanya)

> Sleep and eat. Eat right. Give your body everything you're stripping from it. (Jess, a 29-year-old transgender woman)

> I go to myself, 'Oh God, I'm hanging out to go to sleep', sleep this all off and then I'm back to normal. (Phil)

> With heroin, the next day you've got to have a hit or you're too sick to do anything, you know what I mean? Whereas with speed, the next day it doesn't matter whether you have a hit or not, do you

> know what I'm saying? You still get by, you go to sleep and, you know, you're not sick.
>
> (Bill, 41-year-old man)

Other accounts enacted a collateral reality of addiction as highly complex. In the following interview excerpt, Ryan (51 years old) discusses the psychological aspects of addiction. Earlier in his interview, he described embarking on extended methamphetamine binges lasting several days without sleep or food. He contrasts this youthful bingeing with the more responsibilised agency and subjectivity expressed through, and shaped by, his current 'controlled usage':

> My dealer rang me up last night, because I'm his guinea pig, I give him honest opinions and I'm not using all the time, and he's rung me up last night and asked me to come over and test something in the morning. Well in the old days I would have blown you [the interviewer] off and gone and used but now I feel that I'm a little bit more responsible and I said 'No, I've got an interview'.

In the past, Ryan had chosen methamphetamine over the normative temporal routines of employment, production and deferred gratification. Recently, however, he has become 'a little bit more responsible', attending the research interview as arranged. Whereas NDARC's account of 'compulsive' methamphetamine use in the absence of physical withdrawal emphasises a fixed pathological subject (Chapter 2), Ryan's account emphasises changes in agency, temporality, subjectivity and responsibility – a developmental subject who matures alongside and through his drug use.

Several other interviewees also articulated collateral realities of addiction as a complex phenomenon. For example, when asked about how methamphetamine use impacts on people, Fred (a 22-year-old man) replied:

> The only consistent thing is addiction. So my reasoning is that it is definitely the person and the environment they've grown up in. It's sort of big time the environment, but then the environment produces the person that has an addictive personality and, if they've got nothing good in their life and drugs are the only good thing in their life, then that's the thing they're going to go for more than anything.

Like Fred, Bill enacts a collateral reality of addiction as complexly co-produced by subjects, drugs and contexts:

> I think a lot of people use because they don't have other things in their life, you know, like, they don't have a job or they don't have recreational activities, you know what I mean, to pass the time. And a lot of it's out of boredom.

These collateral realities of addiction depart markedly from the research and policy discourse analysed earlier, in which the health and social problems of methamphetamine addiction arise unilaterally from underlying individual psychology or brain processes. Instead, they offer strikingly nuanced readings, re-asserting the co-production of methamphetamine addiction in experience, subjectivity, and material and discursive contexts.

Another stark difference between the collateral realities enacted in research and policy and those in consumer accounts can be found in the role given to pleasure in narratives of psychological addiction to methamphetamine. Belinda (31 years old) made the following comment about pleasure:

> It's like once you've had your first hit [of methamphetamine] you want another one and then another one after that. Once you come down, you want more and more and more because you just love the feeling, you always want to be like that, there's nothing better. That's what you think and then it just ruins you.

Steve (40 years old) also emphasised pleasure in his account:

> [When I was addicted to speed] it had me by the balls for years. That's why I can't believe I've got to the stage where, you know, because I loved it and I loved it for years and, um, see how I said love. I used to love it, but I used to love, I loved it, because I never got to the – it always had me you know, and that's why even now I don't want to go near it, because if I have a taste... I could fall back in that line [addiction].

Belinda's and Steve's accounts emphasise the pleasure of methamphetamine use, a pleasure that cannot be trusted. They produce methamphetamine as a seductive, malevolent agent – it can 'ruin you' and has its consumers 'by the balls'. In this sense their accounts align with those in research and policy. However, these accounts also constitute pleasure and love in ways that do not map easily onto the reductive certainties of psychological and neuroscientific accounts of addiction. In their focus on subjectivity, emotion and embodiment, these accounts also enact a collateral reality of addiction as co-produced by complex assemblages of subjects, drugs and contexts.

Finally, Phil also enacts methamphetamine addiction, his comments highlighting the potential political effects of addiction treatment discourse. As he puts it, treatment discourse tells us methamphetamine addiction exists even where our own experience tells us it does not:

> Oh apparently, I don't know, it [methamphetamine addiction] exists but I've never experienced it. [...] I've just sort of heard about it, I don't know how I heard about it but oh there's treatments out there or something isn't there? [...] I think I've just sort of heard there's treatments for it so therefore I've assumed that people have been addicted to it or something or they've used it every day for five years so they're addicted to it or something like that.

Here Phil points to the active role of treatment discourse in enacting and sustaining the collateral reality of methamphetamine addiction.

A second aspect of the consumer accounts, one that is highly relevant to the argument we make in this book, is the enactment of a collateral reality in which methamphetamine use is a 'habit' rather than an 'addiction'. Although some participants employed the term as a synonym for 'addiction', others used it in ways that resembled its dictionary definition: that is, as 'a settled or regular tendency or practice, especially one that is hard to give up' (*OED* online version, accessed on 2 August 2013). For example, as Mike said:

> So you can say you're addicted to it [methamphetamine] but scientifically they're going to laugh at you and say it's all in the head, like cigarettes. That's a good example. It's like a cigarette. We're addicted to it but really we're not because if you can get rid of the idea of having a cigarette in your hand and sucking on one, it's really just a habit, not an addiction.

Here Mike offers a rather idiosyncratic reading of scientific understandings of smoking, in the process explicitly defining methamphetamine use not as addiction but as a relatively trivial, routinised bodily and psychological practice. In this sense, Mike's collateral reality of habit constitutes drug use as unexamined, un-reflexive action rather than the outcome of, for example, flawed choice or errant, irremediable brain chemistry.

Jane (23 years old) also invoked the collateral reality of methamphetamine use as habit rather than addiction:

JANE: I see addiction as when you physically can't function without something.

INTERVIEWER: So like heroin where they go into withdrawal?

JANE: Yeah, yeah, so ice, no [it's not addictive] because while it is habit forming it's not physically addictive.

INTERVIEWER: OK, so by habit forming what do you mean?

JANE: Like as in, like, when ice is around you can, like, just say you've got a lot of it in front of you, you might have it in the morning and then you'll have it in the morning and then you'll have it the next morning and the next morning, so it just becomes a habitual part of like your life but it's not addictive to the point where you're physically addicted to it where you, like, you might come down, but you're not like people who come off opiates who have the shakes and then they're going absolutely crazy.

Carl (a 32-year-old man) also drew on the idea of habit to describe cycles of extended consumption followed by extended rest:

> I know I had a habit because I kept using it, but I think it was more a psychological habit than a physical habit, because I never had any withdrawal symptoms. I'd just stop, and by stopping it means you'd either fall asleep where you are, you know, in the car, you'd fall asleep. And someone else gets in and drives and then you wake up a couple of days later in the back seat. [And you wake up and say] 'Yeah, what day is it, what have I missed?' And then, you know, or just getting into bed and you have a good, you know, three days solid sleep, you know? And then you get up, and you're all right. Until the weekend would come, and then they'd all want to do stuff again, and it will all take off like that again.

Likewise, Jess described a period in which she used methamphetamine constantly for two weeks, responding as follows to a question about whether she had experienced paranoia:

JESS: No because I know my limits. I know when it's time to rest.

INTERVIEWER: So even in the two weeks [of constant use]?

JESS: Oh in that two weeks, that was my beginning days of going hard again so, yeah, that's why I stayed up for two weeks, I guess, and the gear was really good.

INTERVIEWER: So do you think that people when they're like that need help or do they just need to have a bit of a lie down?

JESS: Some of them do. Some of them don't realise what their habit has turned [in]to, they can't see anything that's happening.

INTERVIEWER: Do you think there's places [services] that they could go to?

JESS: Oh, there's heaps of places but whether they go or not is another thing.

INTERVIEWER: What would stop them?

JESS: Oh, sometimes nothing until they hit rock bottom. Yeah and even then sometimes that doesn't even help.

Here 'habit' appears again as a routinised bodily practice, albeit one with the potential to become a problem – in the language of 12-step programmes, to 'hit rock bottom'. But this happens only to those who do not realise 'what's happening' – that is, those who are unable or unwilling to interpret their habit through the prism of compulsion or frame it as addiction where necessary.

The interviewees also made frequent references to methamphetamine's effects on the brain. As we have seen in the collateral realities of addiction and habit made in the interviews, participants both reproduce and challenge the collateral realities evident in research and policy – in this case, that of addiction as brain disease, which occupies a more central place in accounts of methamphetamine use than it does in lay accounts of alcohol use (Chapter 5) and of obesity (Chapter 7). The reasons for this difference are likely many, but one obvious one is related to the level of pathologisation of (and thus expert engagement in) different consumption practices, and their impact on target groups. In that drinking alcohol and eating for pleasure are normalised practices in the West, expert health discourse targets individuals in only the most generic and innocuous ways (everyone should eat more fruit and vegetables, moderate their drinking and so on). Consumers of methamphetamine are, by contrast, targeted in highly explicit, highly pathologising ways ('Ice: it's a dirty drug', 'Meth can cause permanent brain damage'). Thus it should come as no surprise that methamphetamine consumers demonstrate an awareness of, and investment in, the prevailing scientific discourses of addiction.

This difference also has other effects. It suggests, for example, that one consequence of the rise of the neuroscience of drugs other than alcohol is a shift to seeing the self as a 'brain' rather than a 'mind'. In the following comment, for example, Rachel (44 years old) offers an explicit (albeit idiosyncratic) neuroscientific explanation for the headaches she used to get after injecting crystalline methamphetamine:

> I'm not medical or anything but in my head I've worked out that, you know, I've fried them fucking little receptors a bit too much and that's why I get a headache. They're not there to cop the rush, so it hurts in other parts of my head.

Other interviews echo the emphasis in research and policy discourse on methamphetamine's capacity to cause hallucinations and delusions, invoking the neuroscience again. For example, Carl said:

> You'd have hallucinations and all that stuff [after using methamphetamine], and your brain was just like fried, like people would have arguments with people on the street, and people would come up to me and say, you know, like, 'Geez, have you heard the word of God?' And I'd be like, 'Of course I have,' you know?

Other consumers also appear to draw on neuroscience in enacting a collateral reality of self as 'brain' rather than 'mind' to explain their decision-making. Consider the following examples:

> I'm an addict – to dope, to speed, to anything I pick up if I pick up the wrong thing. I'm an addict because I smoke every day. I'm an addict because I smoke cigarettes every day as well. I'm an addict because more often than not 'yes' is the answer my brain comes up with and sometimes no matter how fucked I am and I know it's not going to do anything to me I'll just have it anyway so I'm an addict.
>
> (Nicole, 39 years old)

> [People get addicted to methamphetamine] because their brain tells them that they need it. Basically I do because, if your brain is telling you that you need it, even though you're not sick from like when you're having it or whatever, your brain is telling you 'you need it today even though you had it yesterday, the day before, the day before, yeah, you need it today'.
>
> (Tracey, 34 years old)

In these quotations, Nicole and Tracey posit the existence of an agential brain that appears to be divorced from the mind of the knowing subject. Could this be one effect of the constant emphasis on brain structures and chemistry as an explanation for human behaviour – that the brain comes to be seen not as the simultaneous expression of emotion, thought and action but as their agent, or, as a biological antagonist to the 'mind' – the orthodox self who knows what good decisions look like but cannot withstand the brain's power?

In other interviews, consumers offer accounts that emphasise the brain but in ways that do not necessarily mesh with the collateral realities made in research and policy. Like Rachel and Carl, several other interviewees talked about 'fried brains' as a result of methamphetamine use. A possible origin for the term is the infamous Reagan-era, anti-drug public service announcement first aired in 1987 and produced by the Partnership for a Drug-Free America (accessed on 2 August 2013: www.youtube.com/watch?v=nl5gBJGnaXs). The advertisement depicts an egg frying in a pan with the voice-over: 'This is drugs [over an image of cooking oil bubbling in a frying pan]. This is your brain on drugs [an egg is broken, dropped into the oil and begins sizzling]. Any questions?'

Tanya, for example, offers the following explanation of the effects of methamphetamine consumption:

TANYA: I think a lot of people fried their brains sort of doing it that way [using methamphetamine rather than amphetamine].

INTERVIEWER: So what do you mean by 'frying their brains'?

TANYA: Using too much, [the methamphetamine] being too strong, not sleeping, not eating. Not sort of looking after themselves. It didn't matter with me, I ate and I slept.

INTERVIEWER: So what does somebody look like who's fried their brain? Just scattered?

TANYA: Who knows? I mean just being scattered doesn't mean your brain is fried. Not in touch with reality I suppose. I mean I'm not in touch with reality most of the time but that's by choice. I can come back down sort of anytime if you know what I mean.

Although Tanya began by drawing on the fried brain metaphor, with its connotations of neurological damage, she then suggested that people fry their brains when they do not 'look after themselves': in other words, from a combination of drug quantity and strength, and a lack of sleep and food, rather than simply from methamphetamine's effects on the brain. Furthermore, while not being 'in touch with reality' may be characteristic of those with fried brains, for Tanya this state of affairs may also arise from choice.

Suzie (39 years old) also invoked the frying metaphor when she talked about the end of a relationship:

> SUZIE: I used speed for about six or seven years but that ruined my relationship with my partner big time.
>
> INTERVIEWER: What happened?
>
> SUZIE: It [speed] was just frying our brains, constantly frying our brains and [we were] getting paranoid [with] each other, ending up getting violent with each other and stuff like that.
>
> INTERVIEWER: Oh really? Just not trusting the other person or thinking that they'd said something when they didn't?
>
> SUZIE: Yep, all of the above that comes with sleep deprivation.
>
> INTERVIEWER: How long would you go without sleep when you were using the speed?
>
> SUZIE: Oh, days and days and days until you dropped or until you took something that fucking knocked you out.

In this extract, although Suzie describes frying the brain through methamphetamine use as leading to paranoia and violence, she then says they are the result of sleep deprivation. Suzie's account begs an important question that, despite NIDA and others' attempts to stabilise drugs and their effects, remains open in all serious discussions of drugs (as perhaps most vividly demonstrated in emerging discourses of food as drug-like, or in 'behavioural addictions' such as gambling): what is the relationship between brain, drug, the social and the self?

In addition to linking methamphetamine use to hallucinations and delusions, later in his interview Carl used the 'fried brain' metaphor in a different way:

> I've been up too long, so your brain, you know, is fried. So like I was making bad decisions, but like, I didn't do anything, I didn't harm anybody, and like I was just like – she [his girlfriend] was like, 'what should I do?' [to help Carl]. And I'm like, 'I just need to sleep', you know? And so I slept maybe four or five days, you know? And then I was fine again, you know? So I gave it a break for a while.

Here a fried brain leads to poor decision-making which, Carl felt, like Tracey and Suzie, could be remedied simply with sleep.

Later in Suzie's interview, she offered a different definition and account of fried brains, one that seems to blend old and new accounts of the effect of methamphetamine (and of drugs in general) on the brain:

> It [frying your brain] means you take that much of it [methamphetamine] that even the next hit is not doing anything because you've got that much in your system that you don't even feel the next fuckin' rush and that, and yeah, so that's what you call 'fried your brain'. You know it's topping you up, you know that it is topping you up, but you're not getting the rush that you would have, like you did off the first and the second one or whatever, you know, that's 'frying your brain'.

Suzie's account seems closest to neuroscientific accounts of dopamine saturation or depletion, in which extreme intoxication means that taking more of the drug does not produce further increases in noticeable drug effects. In the Australian and NIDA accounts discussed earlier, this is understood as evidence of compulsion. Suzie, however, emphasises a desire to maintain the pleasurable effects of the drug, an aspect of drug use all but invisible in the collateral realities made in these research accounts.

In summary, the collateral realities of addiction enacted in interviews with people who consume methamphetamine both reproduce and challenge those in psychological and neuroscientific research and policy. Although many draw on prevailing collateral realities of addiction by differentiating sharply between 'physical' addiction to opiates and 'psychological' addiction to methamphetamine, their accounts also suggest considerable ambivalence about addiction. Most significantly, whereas the collateral realities enacted in research and policy seek to stabilise addiction ontologically as an anterior and singular entity arising from the brain, and knowable through psychology or neuroscience, consumer accounts undermine this stabilising work and reposition addiction as complex and multiple – as emerging through the co-production of biography, agency, subjectivity, normative expectations, material and discursive resources, pleasure and biomedical discourse. In consumer collateral realities of drug 'habits', methamphetamine use is commonly recuperated from the pathological sphere of 'addiction'. Although sometimes heavy, methamphetamine use is instead constituted as routinised bodily practice – as habit.

Conclusion

In this and the previous chapter, we tracked the enactment of collateral realities of methamphetamine addiction in three discursive realms: research, policy and everyday consumption. Our aim in each case was to understand how these various enactments are remaking addiction and to identify the destabilising gaps, aporias and tensions between these enactments and the realities they perform. In their accounts of the physical sensations of using drugs, of using methamphetamine in the way many people use coffee, of its incorporation into weekend socialising and of its role in 'going hard', consumers of methamphetamine offer alternatives to some of the collateral realities of addiction enacted in research and policy: for example, that methamphetamine dependence and addiction are stable, anterior objects; that they can be reduced to faulty psychology or neurochemistry; that dependence and addiction are unproblematic ways of understanding methamphetamine; that methamphetamine is always and inevitably addictive; and that methamphetamine use is unequivocally harmful. In the Introduction to this book we argued that habit offers a valuable otherwise to addiction, allowing a rather less irredeemably bleak approach to repetition, and scope to bypass the binaries attendant upon addiction – including those that fit very poorly, such as tolerance and withdrawal. As we have seen in this chapter, habit emerges over and over in methamphetamine users' accounts, and it is possible to see how it makes space for rather different engagements than do the realities enacted in research and policy.

That said, consumer accounts of methamphetamine use reproduce as well as challenge the existing research and policy collateral realities of addiction. They incorporate these collateral realities partially and inconsistently – into articulations of addiction, embodiment, pain, time, subjectivity, psychosis, agency, decision-making, responsibility, reality and pleasure. In doing so, they make collateral realities themselves, ones that enact addiction in ways that offer support for our argument in this book: that addiction is made in practice, is only possible in the confluence of complex and emergent phenomena, and proves difficult to stabilise in the multiplicity of its ontological constituents. This, as we will also argue in relation to consumer accounts of alcohol addiction in Chapter 5, is partly right. At the same time that methamphetamine addiction is made in such ontologically multiple ways, many statements are also made that treat it as self-evident and anterior. Methamphetamine addiction has, it seems, many partial enactments, sometimes taken for granted, sometimes subjected to scepticism and critique. As such, we would argue, addiction is dependent not even upon the nature of a substance – this claim is too shallow – but on the particular ontology and epistemology of a substance as it is enacted at a given time and in relation to a given set of circumstances (where circumstances are *part of*, rather than behind, beyond or surrounding the substance). It is, in short, an assemblage.

In the next chapter, we move on to a new section, this time focusing on a substance by turns demonised and entirely normalised: alcohol. In the first of two chapters on alcohol that form this section, we consider the collateral realities of alcohol addiction enacted in sociological, psychiatric, genetic and epidemiological research accounts. In contrast to the vigorous attempts to stabilise methamphetamine use and addiction in research and policy accounts, realities of alcohol addiction have been highly volatile, marked by instability and ambiguity, and subjected to repeated criticism and revision.

4
A Field in Disarray? The Constitution of Alcohol Addiction in Expert Debates

In 1976 Griffith Edwards and Milton Gross published a 'provisional' but extremely influential description of the 'alcohol dependence syndrome' (Edwards & Gross 1976). Since then, alcohol addiction has been heavily contested. In this chapter we continue our analysis of changing definitions and collateral realities of addiction by exploring research on alcohol. In particular, we focus on some of the debates that have constituted and re-constituted alcohol dependence since Edwards and Gross's landmark text, arguing that a concept taken by many to be stable and self-evident is, in expert circles, highly volatile: subjected over and again to criticism, revision and re-definition. This instability and ambiguity mark alcohol addiction out from the methamphetamine addiction found in Chapters 2 and 3 to be so vigorously under stabilisation. How is this difference in the conceptualisation of methamphetamine and alcohol addiction to be explained? There are many possible contributing factors, but perhaps the most obvious are the relatively lengthy history of debate surrounding alcohol compared to the new object of methamphetamine and the widespread and normalised use of alcohol which makes straightforward claims of addiction harder to sustain. If we are to take seriously the role of politics, mores and practices in the constitution of addictions, it follows that as all of these undergo change themselves over time they necessarily help reframe and remake the realities of addiction to which they contribute. As we will argue, it seems that the object long positioned at the heart of concerns about alcohol consumption – addiction – proves, now more than ever, slippery and difficult to stabilise.

Our analysis takes in several debates in which repeated and concerted efforts – in psychiatry, genetics and epidemiology – have been made to stabilise and re-stabilise the elusive object of alcohol addiction. The voluminous literature on alcohol means we had to be selective in our choice of material, but the debates we discuss all exemplify key positions and involve some of the field's leading researchers and institutions. We begin by drawing on some of the work of leading addiction sociologist Robin Room to explore social constructionist work on alcohol addiction. In particular, we highlight the ontological substrate of this work and its consequent struggle to theorise substance, bodies, subjects and practice. Next, we examine the landmark attempt, beginning in the 1970s, to replace the disease of 'alcoholism' with a new psychobiological object – the 'alcohol dependence syndrome'. We then investigate a key site for constituting alcohol addiction as a biological object – genetics (or the 'phenotype' of alcohol addiction). Finally, we continue our discussion of the *DSM*, begun in Chapter 1, by considering contemporary debates over alcohol addiction associated with the development of the *DSM-5* and the subsequent replacement of the 'alcohol dependence syndrome' with yet another stabilised entity – that of 'alcohol use disorder'.

In considering these debates, we ask the following questions in relation to research on alcohol and addiction: What practices – that is, what assemblages of relations – are at work to constitute the realities of alcohol and addiction? How is the stability of these realities achieved and maintained? What collateral realities are being done 'incidentally and along the way' (Law 2011, 156) to aid the achievement and maintenance of stability, and which help to obscure or 'wash away' (Law 2011, 171) this stabilising work? And what gaps, aporias and tensions exist between these practices and the realities they perform? In other words, which collateral realities might offer entry points for destabilising such accounts? Our aim in pursuing these questions is to make visible – and so problematise – the strategic moves undertaken to stabilise various assemblages of alcohol addiction and to draw out their political effects.

The problem of matter: Social constructionist accounts of alcohol addiction

Closely linked with addiction and dependence, alcohol has long interested historians, sociologists and anthropologists. A key theoretical orientation in their work has been that of social constructionism, an approach that focuses on the processes of 'collective definition' involved in constructing 'social problems' such as addiction (Goode & Ben-Yehuda 1994). In this approach social problems do not exist objectively, as is assumed by a positivist epistemology, but are constructed in discourse, practice and politics. Definitions of social problems emerge out of specific sociocultural conditions and structures, operate within particular historical eras and are subject to the influence of particular individuals, social classes and so on. In this section of the chapter, our aim is not to attempt a comprehensive review of the extensive social constructionist literature on alcohol use in general but to trace its specific application to alcohol addiction and dependence in order to provide the conceptual backdrop to our analysis. We do this by considering at length the work of Robin Room, arguably the world's leading sociologist of alcohol use. Room's work, on which we also drew in Chapter 1, both tracks and reflects major stages in sociological scholarship on alcohol. We have chosen this approach on the basis of Room's unparalleled intellectual prominence in and contribution to the field. This is evidenced by the number and extraordinary influence of his qualitative and quantitative sociological publications on alcohol; the many national and international research awards his work has received over the four decades of his output; his leadership role in alcohol and other drug research groups and centres in the United States, Canada, Sweden and Australia; the many senior editorial positions he has occupied with international alcohol and other drug academic journals; and his long-standing advisory work on alcohol issues for the WHO. In short, his work is thoroughly enmeshed in the intellectual and empirical development of the field.

We focus on a series of publications in which Room has both reviewed and contributed (sometimes critically[1]) to the development of social constructionist approaches to alcohol addiction and dependence (Room 1983, 1984b, 1985, 2003). In these works, he explores several of the positions available within the social constructionist tradition as well as advocates a 'soft' constructionism in which the socially constructed concepts of 'alcoholism', 'alcohol addiction' and 'alcohol dependence' are distinct from the reality of biology and pharmacology, which pre-exists and remains ontologically separate from these social constructions.

In a 1983 book chapter, Room pointed to an early social constructionist perspective in considering (mainly North American) sociological contributions to debates on the 'modern alcoholism movement', by which he meant scientific debates occurring in the 1940s–1970s over 'alcoholism's status and characteristics as a disease'. In this movement, Room (1983, 49) argued the ontological position on 'alcoholism' was that it was 'a Platonic entity rather than a human construction; it really exists'. According to Room, the view that

> 'alcoholism is a disease'... includes within it the assertion that alcoholism should be regarded as an entity. In fact, both psychiatric

> and lay discussions which were couched in terms of alcoholism tended not to raise... the issue of the entativity of alcoholism; it was an assumption buried beneath the discussions of exactly how 'it' [alcoholism] was to be defined. (1983, 55)

By comparison, the 'distinctive approach of sociologists... has rather been a nominalist stance to the disease concept – a view of the concept of alcoholism as a social creation of particular times and situations' (Room 1983, 49).

Later in the same piece Room notes how, following the publication of Edwards and Gross's (1976) description of the 'alcohol dependence syndrome' (on which there is more below), a 'bi-axial' conceptualisation of alcohol problems emerged in both scholarly circles and in the policy statements of authoritative bodies such as the WHO. According to Room (1983, 62), this conceptualisation was a 'compromise between clinical and sociological perspectives' and comprised the 'nonentitative (and nondisease) conceptualization' of 'alcohol-related problems' delineating the 'larger territory' of all problems relating to alcohol, whatever their origins and parameters, within which sat a

> diseaselike entity, the 'alcohol dependence syndrome,' including a variety of physical and psychological characteristics, as 'a psychobiological reality, not an arbitrary social label'. (Edwards et al. 1977, 9)

Therefore, while public health epidemiologists and sociologists alike began to focus on the broad range of alcohol-related problems from the late 1970s on, the 'entitative' assumption – the collateral reality of alcohol addiction as an anterior entity – lived on in the alcohol dependence syndrome.

In a 1984 paper, Room again contrasts the 'Platonic idealism which characterizes much clinical thought' on alcoholism with the 'nominalist stance' that has been the 'hallmark of sociological approaches to the disease concept'. But this time, Room argues that:

> Constructivist analyses should resist any tendency to ignore or discount objective realities which act at least as limits on processes of social construction. People die of alcoholic cirrhosis, or in drunken car crashes; others are harmed by the drinker's behavior; a drunken person indeed is less capable of performing skillful tasks. These events are all indeed subject to social construction as to their definition and implications, and the recognition and import of the alcohol

> link, in particular, is subject to construction. But there is still an objective residue, no matter how constructed: the person is dead or harmed, the task undone or done clumsily... [Therefore] the distinctive subject matter of a constructionist sociology of alcohol problems... [is] the interaction between these processes [of problem definition] and objective conditions... [that is] the dialectic between social definitions and material circumstances. (1984b, 9–10)

In other words, there are social constructions and there is an anterior objective reality, and the two should be seen as ontologically separate.

In an article in the *British Journal of Addiction* (Room 1985), Room considers three ways in which sociocultural contexts can be taken into account in understanding alcohol dependence. The first stance is 'simply to take dependence or addiction as a given...and to consider psychosocial among other factors in its occurrence' (133). Within this perspective, the prevalence of alcohol dependence is 'affected by [correlated with or caused by] sociocultural factors'. The second stance involves deconstructing the ' "given," the disease or condition or dependent variable, and to consider to what extent sociocultural factors can be part of the essence of what is to be explained' (1985, 133). The third – 'constructivist' or 'historical social constructionist' – stance is to 'distance ourselves from the disease or condition or dependent variable, and so shift to the question of how such conceptions as the disease concept of alcoholism or addiction arise' – in other words, to regard the addiction concept as a 'sociocultural creation that tells us as much about structures of thought in a given social order as about the nature or reality of individual experience' (1985, 133). This perspective 'takes one step further back from the comfortable platonic positivism' by viewing the 'dependence concept itself' as a 'sociocultural construction, located in a particular time and place and sociocultural circumstances' (1985, 134).

Taking up this third, constructionist, stance, Room offers an analysis in which he zeroes in on the central aspect of dependence – its 'pathognomic symptom' (Room 1985, citing Jellinek 1952) – 'loss of control'. Reviewing key works in sociology (Lemert 1951), history (McCormick 1969; Levine 1978) and anthropology (Kunitz & Levy 1974; Leland 1976), Room concludes that:

> In the context of American and British societies, then, it can be argued that both the idea of addiction and existential experience of loss of control to which the idea refers are historical creations

> of a particular epoch, reflecting a particular organization of society. (1985, 136)

However, he is also careful to state that in conceptualising alcohol addiction or dependence in this way – as 'culture-bound' – he is not 'denying the transcultural reality of the withdrawal syndrome or other physical accompaniments and sequelae of heavy or prolonged drinking'. Instead, Room draws attention to those

> aspects that have usually fallen under the rubric of 'psychological dependence'. In my view, looked at in cross-cultural perspective, it is questionable whether these necessarily covary with the physical accompaniments or sequelae of drinking... therefore, it would be unwise to assume that the various elements described as the 'alcohol dependence syndrome' constitute a single 'psychobiological reality'... rather, variations in the sociocultural construction of drinking behavior – dependence concepts and experiences, as well as other concepts and experiences – should be made the subject of empirical investigation, along with studies of the sociocultural patterning and biological concomitants of drinking. (1985, 137)

In other words, Room separates the pharmacological 'reality' of alcohol as a material substance, and the 'transcultural reality' of alcohol's effects on human biology, from socially constructed concepts and experiences. In this sense, Room's position is close to that of MacAndrew and Edgerton (1969), and also of Marshall (1979, 1) who argued that '[t]he cross-cultural study of alcohol presents a classic natural experiment: a single species (*Homo sapiens*), a single drug substance (ethanol), and a great diversity of behavioral outcomes'. In this formulation, we see the enactment of a collateral reality of addiction in which human biology and the substance of alcohol are positioned as universal constants, and sociocultural and historical contexts are positioned as varying according to time and place.

In 'The cultural framing of addiction' (Room 2003), Room again takes up these issues:

> We are not concerned here with the truth value of addiction and cognate terms or with their empirical applicability. Thus we are not concerned, for instance, with whether there is really a single entity called 'alcoholism' or whether alcoholism is really a disease. Instead, the concern is with what is meant when we talk about addiction and

> with the ways in which this conceptualization of behavior and events may be culturally framed. (2003, 221)

In this paper, he re-traces the argument that a central feature of the addiction concept – loss of control or impaired control – is culturally framed, but he also adds two further cultural elements. The first is that (malign) agency is often located in the drug in question and causal links are made between ingestion of the drug and 'bad behaviour'. The second is that assessments of negligence regarding the fulfilment of responsibilities and obligations on the part of addicted or dependent persons rely heavily on culturally specific temporal norms, a point we also made earlier about the *DSM-5* criteria (see Chapter 1). Here, Room's paper again enacts biology as distinct from culture. Withdrawal from alcohol ('the physical and psychological discomforts that often occur when use of a drug is ceased and that can usually be relieved by further use of the drug') and tolerance ('[t]here is no doubt about the existence of the various phenomena lumped together as tolerance') are universal features of human biology even if their meanings are to a large extent culturally determined.

In the final section of the 2003 article, Room adds an important caveat to his argument about the conferral of meaning:

> Let me make clear that my argument does not amount to an attempt to explain away addiction. Nor, in particular, would I want to deny the experience of the many thousands of people in American society and elsewhere who have felt that they could not control their drinking or drug use and thus their lives. For many, addiction and related concepts have both given them a way of understanding their experience and also has been of therapeutic value. To argue that a concept is culturally constructed and framed is not to argue that it is wrong or useless. (2003, 232)

Like Room's earlier statements, we see his insistence on two components to addiction: a subjective reality, which is made and re-made in cultural practice, and an anterior reality (perhaps biological to judge by his earlier insistence on the transcultural reality of alcohol's pharmacological effect on human bodies) beneath and beyond cultural construction and meaning making. But he goes a step further than simply maintaining this distinction here, in arguing that drawing attention to the cultural framing of addiction does not mean that addiction is 'wrong or useless'. But if addiction as cultural reality is not wrong, does that mean it is right? And in what sense can we say it is right if it is indeed a cultural framing located in a specific place and time? The problem here is the collateral reality the article enacts in which material (biological, pharmacological) substance is separated from cultural practice. We return to this conceptual problem below.

Room's critical analyses, and those of the historians, sociologists and anthropologists he cited, were crucial conceptual interventions in an era dominated by the governing image of 'alcoholism' (Room 2001). They served to undermine taken-for-granted ideas about alcohol addiction built on entitative disease assumptions and drew attention to the cultural dimension of addiction. Room's work goes a step further than many constructionist accounts which, in seeking to escape biological determinism and emphasise reality as exclusively shaped by history and culture, neglect the role of materiality. But, working within a particular theoretical paradigm, Room reintroduced a 'dialectic between social definitions and material [e.g. biological, pharmacological] circumstances' (Room 1984b, 10). Thus, while the *concepts* of 'alcoholism', 'alcohol addiction' and 'alcohol dependence' are socially constructed and framed, the *reality* of material circumstances, of biology and pharmacology, pre-exists and remains ontologically separate from these constructions.

Such perspectives prompt a series of questions. Are there irrefutable biological facts with which we can generalise about alcohol addiction, or are the biological aspects of alcohol addiction usefully seen as themselves socially constituted? Could it be that there is no fixed reality beyond that posited, defined and disseminated by social constructions, by the production of knowledges? Surely not. For many, reality is, in the last instance, defined by matter. Are social constructionists going too far in emphasising the role of culture and society in the production of reality? Do theoretically elegant ideas about reality being socially constituted fail in the face of the biological 'facts'? Who would want to dismiss, for example, liver cirrhosis as merely a discursive construction, as if a change in ways of talking and thinking about it would alter it or instantly prevent it from happening? How can we acknowledge the role of materiality in the production of realities without characterising that role as determining? Rather than embracing one or other of the positions available in the social constructionist work explored and exemplified by Room, in this chapter (and in this book as a whole) we draw instead on recent work in STS to examine research on alcohol addiction in a new way. We turn to this work because it offers a way out of Room's impasse by recognising that material objects – such as alcohol – are neither purely the product of social practices nor entirely determined by their supposedly intrinsic material attributes. Instead, people, objects and concepts make and remake each other in specific encounters, and continue to do so for as long as such encounters occur.

As we noted earlier, Room highlighted the impact of the publication of Edwards and Gross's (1976) description of the 'alcohol dependence syndrome' on research and policy. In the next sections, we explore the practices at work since 1976 to constitute the reality of alcohol dependence. How is the stability of alcohol dependence achieved and maintained, if indeed it is, and what realities made 'along the way' support the achievement and maintenance of this stability? What strategic moves are evident in this stabilisation and what are their political effects? And which collateral realities might offer entry points for destabilising such accounts?

Stabilising the 'alcohol dependence syndrome'

In 1976, psychiatrists Griffith Edwards and Milton Gross published a landmark article entitled 'Alcohol dependence: Provisional description of a clinical syndrome' (Edwards & Gross 1976). In doing so, they acknowledged that theirs was 'far from the first attempt to describe the syndrome', with 'Jellinek's classification of alcoholism into types stand[ing] supreme' (Edwards & Gross 1976, 1058). Ten years later, Edwards (1986) published a second article – 'The alcohol dependence syndrome: A concept as stimulus to enquiry' – in which he summarised research on the alcohol dependence syndrome stimulated by the publication of the 1976 article. This work has continued to shape research, policy and practice in the alcohol field ever since (informing, for example, the development of the WHO's *International Classification of Diseases* and the American Psychiatric Association's *DSM*). As we show later in the chapter, however, the addiction object stabilised in these two publications – the 'alcohol dependence syndrome' – has been the subject of extensive revision via genetics and epidemiology as attempts have arisen to stabilise new alcohol problem objects.

We argue that the reality of the 'alcohol dependence syndrome' was constituted and stabilised through the following collateral realities, all of which are enacted at various points in the two publications:

- clinical knowledge and the need to treat problem drinkers require new ways of framing alcoholism;

- dependence constitutes a definite 'syndrome' that can be treated despite its description remaining 'provisional';
- dependence is an ontologically anterior 'pathological process';
- the various aspects of this pre-constituted object can be identified through multidisciplinary research; and
- environments are external to the 'psychobiological core' of dependence.

As we show, the alcohol dependence syndrome remakes alcohol addiction as a clinical problem that needs to be addressed through treatment, enacts medicine as a suitable epistemological frame and locates addiction within the pathological drinker.

The first collateral reality we identify is an epistemological one to do with the role of clinical knowledge and the need to treat problem drinkers in providing both the justification and evidence for the development of a new way of framing alcoholism. As Edwards and Gross (1976, 1058) put it: 'Anyone concerned with treating drinking problems must find that his [*sic*] patient often tells him more than is in the textbooks.' In the 1986 article, which reviewed research stimulated by the publication of the 1976 article, Edwards repeats the claim that the key aim of clinical research and practice is to understand 'how the individual may be treated and drinking problems prevented'. In this way, as we argued in relation to amphetamine dependence in Chapters 2 and 3, alcohol addiction must be stabilised in order that policy and practice can respond effectively. This concern for improving the treatment of drinking problems underpins Edwards and Gross's aim to 'delineate the clinical picture' of the 'alcohol dependence syndrome – a condition far better described by the average alcoholic than in any book'. While acknowledging their laudable concern for the plight of the 'average alcoholic', readers might also be struck by their apparent confidence. Indeed, an alternative and equally plausible rendering of their concern might run as follows: 'There seems to be some kind of problem with alcohol that differs from previous understandings of alcoholism. We do not know what this problem is, and we do not really understand it or even know if it exists, but we desperately need to treat it.'

In the quotation cited in the previous paragraph, Edwards and Gross do not define what they mean by the 'average alcoholic'. But he or she is then enrolled in the task of helping to construct a new understanding of alcoholism, even as Edwards and Gross acknowledge that the application of such a term, and the exposure of 'alcoholics' to existing treatment regimes, enrols them in a discourse producing specific forms of subjectivity, agency and pathology (Bourgois 2000; Ning 2005; Moore 2009). As Edwards and Gross note:

> Routine clinical questions may impose a pattern on patients' accounts, and patients may themselves organise their uncertain recall of events in terms of expectations given to them. (1976, 1058)

While Edwards and Gross are, it seems, aware of the circularity of policy and treatment discourse that assumes the phenomenon it seeks to define, measure and address, they demonstrate some difficulty extracting their own work from this cycle.

The second, related, collateral reality made in the two publications is that dependence constitutes a definite 'syndrome' that can be treated despite its description remaining 'provisional'. In the 1976 article, Edwards and Gross concede that attempting a 'definitive description of this syndrome is premature' and that 'much is still only at the stage of "clinical impression"'. This emphasis on the 'provisional', impressionistic nature of their description, also evident in the article's title, re-appears throughout the 1976 and 1986 articles. Yet they claim that the 'clinical impression' they offer is underpinned by the 'psychobiological basis of dependence' (on which more below). They go on to outline seven 'essential elements of the syndrome', again, however, qualifying their stabilising move by describing their list of elements as only 'provisionally' including

> a narrowing in the repertoire of drinking behaviour; salience of drink-seeking behaviour; increased tolerance to alcohol; repeated withdrawal symptoms; repeated relief or avoidance of withdrawal symptoms by further drinking; subjective awareness of a compulsion to drink; [and] reinstatement of the syndrome after abstinence. (1976, 1058)

The awkward juxtaposition of 'essential' and 'provisional' elements continues when they state that not all of these elements 'need always be present, nor always present with the same intensity' (1976, 1058). Within the authors' attempt at provisional stabilisation, then, lies a tension over consistency and variation. What, we might ask, defines the alcohol dependence syndrome if all elements need not be present – that is, if different drinkers exhibit different subsets of the seven elements?[2] Further complicating the picture is their insistence that, irrespective of the severity and/or accumulation of these elements for specific individuals, they all relate to an 'underlying psychobiological process'.

Edwards and Gross conclude the 1976 article by suggesting that

> a clinical syndrome of alcohol dependence can now be recognised fairly confidently... Very speculatively, we may suppose that... the abnormality involves both a biological process and aberrant learning... [alcohol] dependence should perhaps be seen as being in the same group of disorders as phobic and obsessional states, with a potent, complicating biological factor. (1061)

Further evidence that the caution implied by the term 'provisional' is not to be taken seriously appears in the 1976 article when Edwards and Gross (1976, 1061) set out an ambitious future research programme predicated on the syndrome's existence: 'one important priority is the sharper delineation of the actual syndrome and of its natural histories [i.e., the "evolution of a pathological process"] and social settings... [and] determining piece by piece the psychobiological basis [of dependence]'.

Later, although Edwards does not exactly 'wash away' (Law 2011) the assumptions and mechanisms by which the reality of alcohol dependence is stabilised, he does proceed as though these assumptions and mechanisms have little or no practical salience:

> [W]ith all due warnings about limitation and time-boundedness born in mind (and the word 'provisional' again underlined), the alcohol dependence syndrome has the potential to act as a much needed stimulus to jolt us out of a bored and unconstructive circling around old positions... (1986, 172)

And:

> Having considered all the evidence... what can we fairly (but provisionally) conclude? With all the proper reservations as to the imperfection of instruments, shortcomings in statistical methods, sampling bias and difficulties with this or that individual piece of research, it would require a certain amount of boldness to dismiss the alcohol dependence syndrome as no more than a chimera. (1986, 180)

Edwards, indeed, concludes:

> The research that we have summarized shows that over the last few years the syndrome concept has catalyzed a range of productive contributions coming from many different centres. The syndrome formulation begins to look like a 'useful idea'. (1986, 181)

This rather modest (and possibly disingenuous) claim ignores the influence of the alcohol dependence syndrome spelt out in 1976 on the development of both the WHO's *International Classification of Diseases* and the American Psychiatric Association's *DSM-III* and *DSM-IV*. What was presented as a 'provisional description', a 'clinical impression' and a 'useful idea' became the basis for the two most widely used international screening instruments for the diagnosis, classification and management of those deemed to have drinking problems.

Evident in some of the above quotations is the third collateral reality to which we wish to attend – the production of alcohol dependence as an 'abnormality', a pathological process or entity that pre-exists the various scientific attempts to define and understand it. This view is also evident in the first collateral reality we noted above – that alcohol addiction requires clarification in order to improve its treatment, with the 1976 and 1986 articles representing early steps in an epistemological journey dedicated to gaining clearer insight into this 'condition'. It is also clear in the following quotation taken from the end of the 1976 article: 'the person who has become dependent on alcohol is certainly ill; and the possibility of contracting this illness awaits anyone who drinks very heavily' (Edwards & Gross 1976, 1061). Perhaps the starkest example of the anterior status of dependence is provided by the following passage from Edwards' 1986 article:

> [O]ne of the most constant problems with our attempts to understand the nature of alcoholism is the feeling that we go around in circles, that inebriety, the disease theory, gamma alcoholism, call it what you will, are lost and rediscovered, 'socially constructed', dismembered and put together again. (1986, 172)

Although conceding that '[u]nderstanding of the nature of this condition is still incomplete', he further claims that 'research has now reached a stage where it is legitimate to go beyond the question as to whether a dimensional syndrome exists, to an exploration of theoretical questions relating to its scientific basis'. In both these passages,

Edwards figures alcohol addiction as an entitative 'it' (Room 1983) that has so far eluded scientific understanding but lies waiting to be revealed.

Having established that the pathological syndrome of alcohol dependence exists, Edwards moves on to enact a fourth collateral reality – that the various aspects of this pre-constituted object can be identified through multidisciplinary research. As he explains, 'Further elucidation will require contributions from many different disciplines' (1986, 171). In inviting contributions from other disciplines (which ones does he mean – feminist theory? history? sociology?), the invitation comes with a serious string attached – those invited must agree to further elucidate a syndrome already established as psychobiological by clinical practice. Here, in entering a 'plea... for a spirit of openness and interdisciplinary enquiry rather than perseveration with the unproductive rhetoric of the "disease" debate' (1986, 171), Edwards acknowledges but then sidelines the various sociological critiques of the alcohol dependence syndrome such as that by Shaw (1979), who argued that the syndrome was merely the disease concept repackaged to meet the various challenges to the medical hegemony of 'alcoholism'.

Indeed, Edwards' response in the 1986 article to Shaw's (1979) criticism is extremely informative. He acknowledges Shaw's key claim – that the alcohol dependence syndrome was a 'substitute concept – one which coped with all the critiques of the disease theory of alcoholism, yet which retained all its major assumptions and implications' – and its political effect – to retain 'medical hegemony'. He describes it as a 'provocative' analysis but one which 'needs to be tested against a more complete historical analysis'. He then traces what he sees as the two key factors in the 'genesis of the dependence syndrome': the emphasis on psychological learning theories, and the application of 'clinical experience which encouraged exact observation'. In offering this historical background, Edwards attempts to dismiss Shaw's allegation that the alcohol dependence syndrome was developed in order to retain 'medical hegemony', but several questions remain about his account. The clinical experience to which Edwards refers is psychiatric in nature, and medical practitioners would surely have been aware of the psychosomatic component in the aetiology of disease and illness. Furthermore, Edwards and Gross employ several terms with distinct medical overtones throughout the 1976 article that is the subject of Shaw's critique: 'condition', 'symptoms', 'natural history', 'illness' and – most significantly given their desire to escape the conceptual baggage of 'alcoholism' – 'disease'. Having offered this unconvincing rebuttal of Shaw's key points, Edwards concludes his response thus: 'The projection of old conflicts about the disease concept onto the dependence formulation is unlikely to be helpful' (1986, 174).

With Shaw's sociological critique summarily dismissed, Edwards re-states the existence of the syndrome and carefully delineates the questions open to multidisciplinary investigation:

> We would seem now to have reached a stage where it is legitimate and indeed vital to start addressing the theoretical issues. What are the processes and mechanisms which lead to the establishment of this condition, maintain its dynamic once it is established, lead to its easy reinstatement after a period of abstinence, or sometimes allow its reversal or extinction? The advantage of the syndrome concept is that it invites the multidisciplinary exploration of this range of questions whereas essentially arbitrary classification systems such as that offered by DSM III cannot have the same heuristic significance. (1986, 181)

In other words, the collateral reality of multidisciplinarity championed by Edwards welcomes diverse contributions as long as they accept the existence of the alcohol dependence syndrome, refrain from criticism of its medical overtones and are content to research its establishment, dynamism and reinstatement or extinction. At best, this seems a very superficial view of multidisciplinarity; at worst, it is multidisciplinarity in name only.

The final collateral reality enacted in the two publications is the conceptual positioning of the socio-cultural or the environment as external to the syndrome. Towards the end of the 1986 article, Edwards offers the following framework:

> The dependence syndrome is a concept which is rooted in psychological, biological and socio-cultural constructs, and which therefore invites no one 'level of explanation' nor the hegemony of any scientific discipline. (1986, 181)

Here, in keeping with his constitution of the collateral reality of multidisciplinary research, the socio-cultural component is given equal weight to the psychological and biological.

Earlier in the article, however, and also in the 1976 one, Edwards defines dependence as an internal condition with a psychobiological basis. Whereas the 'ordinary drinker's consumption' is 'patterned by varying internal cues and external circumstances', the 'dependent person begins to drink the same whether it is work day, weekend, or holiday: the nature of the company or his [*sic*] own mood makes less and less difference' (Edwards & Gross 1976, 1058). In this scheme, the psychobiological core of dependence can be 'shaped and coloured' – can be constrained or liberated – by 'personality and environment' but is conceptualised as a distinct, discrete process internal to the individual. In the 1976 article, Edwards and Gross offer a similarly individualised framing:

> What happens to the dependent person is determined not only by the progression of a disease but also by social processes. These help determine the rate of development of the syndrome, the secondary consequencies [*sic*], the help offered, the degree of stigmatisation. (1976, 1060)

Here, the 'dependent person' is a pre-constituted subject whose diseased condition improves or worsens according to the impact of external social processes.

Putting together the collateral realities enacted in these two works on the alcohol dependence syndrome, we find that

- addiction to alcohol can be identified clinically and this is necessary for better treatment;
- an addiction syndrome can be both provisional and a definite basis for action;
- alcohol addiction exists anterior to its investigation;
- multidisciplinary research can help to delineate alcohol addiction but only if it accepts a medical view of this condition; and
- the environment is secondary and external to the internal psychobiological core of addiction.

These collateral realities remake alcohol addiction as a clinical problem that needs to be addressed through treatment, as an entitative 'it' (Room 1983) rather than a 'provisional' syndrome, as knowable primarily through the guiding epistemological frame of medicine, and as located within a pre-constituted pathological subject. But even as this stable reality was being established, researched and promulgated, another version of alcohol addiction was already looming on the scientific horizon – that of alcohol addiction as genetic.

From past to present: Stabilising alcohol addiction as genetic

As they have for every other key social and political issue, new technologies have raised fresh questions on the nature of addiction and reopened old ones. In this section, we analyse research attempts to redefine and stabilise alcohol addiction via genetics, a field which is also neuroscientific in its orientation. Genetic studies of alcohol use often focus on neurotransmitters, so it is unclear which are 'genetic studies' and which qualify for the description 'neuroscience'. Work on the alcohol dependence syndrome discussed in the previous section emphasised a psychobiological core underpinning alcohol addiction but left open the challenge of 'determining piece by piece [this] psychobiological basis' (Edwards & Gross 1976, 1061). Genetic and neuroscientific research has enthusiastically taken up this challenge, locating addiction in the narrowly biological brain and body. We examine four reviews on alcohol published in *Addiction*, the highest-ranked international, generalist journal in the field. Two of these articles were published in *Addiction*'s 'Horizons Review' series, one in the 'Addiction and its Sciences' series and one under the general heading of 'Review', another regular section of the journal. These reviews provide extensive summaries of recent and emerging developments in genetic approaches to alcohol addiction – authored by researchers based in the Netherlands, the United Kingdom and the United States. Two of the articles (Agrawal & Lynskey 2008; Ball 2008) examine recent research on the genetic basis of addiction in general but devote considerable space to alcohol-specific research. The other two articles (Ducci & Goldman 2008; Van der Zwaluw & Engels 2009) specifically examine recent scientific literature on alcohol. Taken together, the reviews argue that alcohol problems have a significant genetic component and can be addressed by future biomedical interventions that draw on gene therapies.

We argue that these review articles attempt to constitute and stabilise a new reality of alcohol addiction. They do so by enacting the following collateral realities of alcohol dependence:

- addiction is an ontologically anterior entity that exists independently of the specific terms used to define it;
- the 'problem' of alcohol encompasses virtually all alcohol use;
- 'environment' can be measured and linked to specific genes;
- the many limitations of genetic evidence can be ignored; and
- science will eventually uncover the reality of alcohol addiction.

Although there are continuities with the collateral realities enacted by Edwards and Gross (for example, that dependence is an ontologically anterior entity), genetic approaches refine their conclusions to move alcohol dependence more explicitly into a biomedical space.

The first noteworthy aspect of the review articles that strikes even the casual reader is the wide variety of terms used, often in the same article (and even in the same sentence or paragraph), to identify the object of study. For example, Ball (2008), in a review article entitled 'Addiction science and its genetics', begins with numerous references to 'addiction'. But when referring specifically to alcohol, the relevant designations become without explanation 'alcohol-related problems', 'dependence' and 'alcoholism'. Agrawal and Lynskey (2008) refer to 'addictive disorders', 'addictive diseases', 'alcohol dependence', 'alcoholism', 'alcohol problems/dependence' and 'alcohol abuse/dependence'. Ducci and Goldman (2008) open their review article by defining 'alcohol use disorders' as 'common and etiologically complex diseases' and alcohol as an 'addictive drug', but, perhaps reflecting their institutional location in the US National Institute on Alcohol Abuse and Alcoholism (NIAAA), favour the term 'alcoholism', which they then use throughout their article. Van der Zwaluw and Engels (2009) are even less precise. They review studies incorporating 'gene-environment interactions in examining alcohol use or dependence in humans' and in other sections of the article describe their focus as 'alcohol (ab)use' and 'alcohol abuse or dependence'. They also note that 'molecular genetic research has described a number of candidate genes that might be associated with susceptibility for alcohol consumption and dependence' (Van der Zwaluw & Engels 2009, 907).

What can we make of the deployment of this dazzling array of terms? What collateral realities are being enacted in this multiplying nomenclature? First, in the absence of definitions of the terms and their referents,[3] we can conclude that the 'problem' of alcohol (whether it be denoted by 'alcoholism', 'dependence', 'disorder', 'disease' or some other term) does not, in the authors' eyes, require exact specification. Instead, this terminological multiplicity, through its very lack of precision, helps to stabilise an ontologically anterior object – in the language we have encountered so far in this and previous chapters, a 'pathological process', 'syndrome', 'disease', 'condition' or 'illness' (Edwards & Gross 1976), a 'real beast' or 'state' (Edwards 1980), an 'it' (Edwards 1986) or an 'entity' (Room 1983) – an elusive but broad biological reality that awaits discovery as new genetic research technologies, methods and findings emerge.

The second collateral reality being enacted through the deployment of multiple, overlapping terms for alcohol addiction has to do with researchers' interest in the scope of the 'problem'. What forms of alcohol consumption, we must ask, remain unquestioned, remain beyond the orbit of genetics, when the area of research interest is defined as alcohol 'use', 'consumption', 'dependence', 'abuse', 'problems', 'alcoholism' and 'human alcohol outcomes'? Such designations cover all drinking, regardless of rates, amounts, frequency and consumption practices. In the alcohol and other drug field more generally, these terms are widely understood as relating to, or describing, very different modes of drinking. 'Alcohol use' and 'human alcohol outcomes' can obviously refer to all alcohol consumption, even that occurring in the absence of 'problems' such as addiction. 'Alcohol abuse' and 'problems' generally refer to acute forms of harm, such as accidents or violence, that do not necessarily involve addiction, with the latter term also being used as an umbrella term for all forms of alcohol-related harm, whether acute or chronic. As explained in the previous section, 'alcohol dependence' has been established to refer to a psychobiological process characterised by compulsion, tolerance and withdrawal. 'Alcoholism', as we noted in an earlier endnote, generally refers to a 'chronic relapsing disorder' or a disease condition. Here, the multiple possible assemblages of substance, bodies, subjects and practice are eclipsed and the many engagements with, and problems related to, alcohol brought within the purview of alcohol addiction, a move that allows greater numbers of drinkers to be pathologised, and more terrain on which geneticists may do their work.

The third collateral reality made in genetic research on alcohol addiction relates to the question of 'environment' or the 'context of addiction'. All four reviews include at least some discussion of the environment, and the interaction between genes and environment is Van der Zwaluw and Engels' main focus (2009). All simplify 'environment' in some way and this simplification is necessary in this context because alcohol addiction is often rendered as a 'phenotype' – a stable object consisting of the observable behavioural characteristics or traits of the 'condition' suffered by an affected person – with research aiming to link the phenotype with specific genes, 'environmental factors' or 'variables', or 'gene–environment interactions'.

The first key way in which environment is simplified is by treating culturally specific, complex and/or politically charged phenomena as singular, settled and uncontroversial 'variables', 'factors' or 'influences'. Examples of such variables include 'conduct disorder', 'depression', 'childhood adversity', 'maltreatment' and personality traits such as 'impulsive sensation seeking' (Ball 2008). Van der Zwaluw and Engels (2009) discuss the role of 'adverse environments', 'environmental risk factors', 'environmental stressors' and even 'environmental pathogens', and give as examples 'negative or inadequate parenting', 'bad parenting', 'poor family relations', 'quality of family relations' and 'maltreatment'. For 'behavioural childhood measures', they list 'impulsivity, self-control, conduct problems and aggression' as 'early [environmental] predictors of heavy alcohol use, alcohol-related problems and dependence later in life' (Van der Zwaluw & Engels 2009, 911).[4] Of course, these terms refer not to objective conditions or states of affairs but to assemblages of relations, concepts and objects held in place through complex historical and political processes involving the medicalisation of deviance (Conrad & Schneider 1992) and the rise of the modern, self-governing subject heralded in part by the rise of the psy disciplines (Rose 1989). Having been established by science, they are treated as simply and self-evidently real.

Agrawal and Lynskey's (2008) review provides another example of the simplification of environment. Reviewing the findings of a set of adoption studies, they state that 'genetic and environmental risk mechanisms operate similarly across genders', and they highlight the 'etiological importance' of 'parental divorce' as a risk factor for alcohol and other drug 'abuse' (Agrawal & Lynskey 2008, 1070). While the first statement is of course hard to credit when one considers the many decades of feminist research on the gendering of bodies and subjectivities and recent theorising on the politics and performativity of gender (see, for example, Butler 1990, 1993), and in turn the very different rates of alcohol consumption for men and women, it is the second statement concerning the aetiological role of divorce that is most striking here. Adopting, even as the article attempts an objective review, a notably conservative political stance, it valorises the role of the nuclear (un-divorced or 'intact') family as protection against 'drug abuse'.

A third key way in which 'environment' is simplified in genetic studies is to treat it as equivalent to the 'family'. For example, Ball (2008, 360) sets out to summarise the 'current and complex view... that multiple genes interact with environmental factors at different stages during the development of addiction'. Instead, his review focuses in large part on family, twin and adoption studies. About adoption studies he makes the following claim: 'These natural experiments transport a high-risk individual from the assumed predisposing environmental influence of the affected biological parent to a novel and potentially protective adoptive environment' (Ball 2008, 361). Here, 'environment' is equated with the influence of a single biological parent (are all of the adopted children from single-parent families – already defined as deviating from the norm of two parents – or are these families in which only one or other biological parent is defined to be an 'alcoholic'?) or the protection afforded by the adoptive family (the political stance here is of the adoptive family as normal). No definition of family is provided, and no acknowledgement is made of different cultural definitions of what constitutes 'family' or of the unusualness of adoption. Rather, the concept is naturalised as pertaining to the nuclear Western family with the single parent as the deviant, and therefore blameworthy, form.

Ducci and Goldman provide a particularly stark rendering of environment as reducible to family:

> Alcoholism occurs due to individual choice, environmental and genetic determinants and interactions between factors within these three domains of causation... Environmental factors include alcohol availability, parental attitudes, peer pressure, underage drinking and childhood maltreatment. (2008, 1418)

Here, 'individual choice' is treated as conceptually distinct from 'environmental and genetic determinants'. Ducci and Goldman's diagram of the 'main and interactive effects of genetic and environmental risk factors for alcoholism' is reproduced below (Figure 4.1).

The diagram consists of three parts: an 'environment' circle, a 'gene' circle and a 'mediating factors' box. The 'risk factors' listed inside the 'environment' circle are 'maternal psychopathology',[5] 'parental alcoholism', 'harsh inconsistent discipline', 'parental rejection' and 'physical and sexual abuse'. Inside the 'gene' circle are the abbreviated names of seven specific genes (for example, 'MAOA' [monoamine oxidase A], 'ALDH2' [aldehylde dehydrogenase 2]). Inside the 'mediating factors' box are listed 'alcohol availability', 'emotional and social support', 'peer influences' and 'socio-economic status'. In this diagram, and contrary to the associated text, 'environment' is enacted as 'family' whereas aspects of the external world (licensing regulations concerning alcohol, socio-economic status and so on) that social science usually treats as 'environmental' are treated as 'mediating factors' between the family environment and genetic endowment.[6]

What can we make of this treatment of environment? One possible answer is that simplifying environment to a limited set of singular, settled and uncontroversial factors or variables, or to the internal dynamics of families, is consistent with a contemporary neo-liberal discourse that

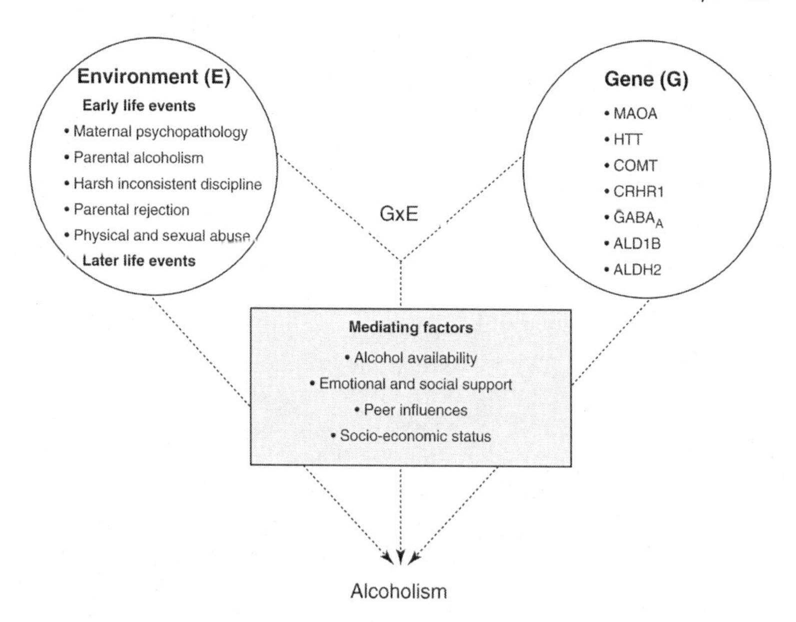

Figure 4.1 Main and interactive effects of genetic and environmental risk factors for alcoholism

valorises independent, autonomous actors who freely exercise individual choice. Framed this way, the treatment of environment in genetic research produces alcohol addiction as either an individual problem of unregulated conduct and genes or a problem of family dysfunction and genes. Both seem more amenable to interventions inspired by neo-liberalism than would be complex, seemingly intractable issues such as marginalisation and structural disadvantage (Moore & Fraser 2006).

The fourth collateral reality enacted in genetic research on alcohol addiction concerns the treatment of evidence, particularly that relating to causation. Do genes, or the interaction between genes and environment, cause alcohol addiction? Or are they best understood as contributing factors? The reviews adopt contradictory positions on this crucial issue. Although their aim is to 'advance our knowledge of the genetic bases of alcoholism', Ducci and Goldman (2008) investigate genetic factors for 'liability' or 'vulnerability' to 'alcoholism and related phenotypes' rather than for 'alcoholism' per se. The focus for Agrawal and Lynskey (2008), identified in the opening line of their abstract, is also the 'genetic basis for addiction', but their article is entitled 'genetic influences on addiction'. In the article itself, they write of 'heritable influences on liability to drug abuse/dependence' and of 'genes conferring susceptibility to addictive diseases' within the context of 'establishing that genetic influences are important etiological factors for addiction'. The use of 'etiology' implies causation: it is the aspect of medicine that is concerned with the origins of disease and illness. The subtle change in language from 'genetic basis' to 'genetic influence' is also interesting. 'Base' is 'the lowest part or edge of something, especially the part on which it rests or is supported... a conceptual structure or entity on which something draws or depends... a main or important element or ingredient to which other things are added' (*OED* online version, accessed on 21 June 2013). However, 'influence' is defined as 'the capacity to have an effect on the character, development, or behaviour of someone or something, or the effect itself' (*OED* online version, accessed on 21 June 2013). Whereas 'base' is foundational, 'influence' is a capacity of pre-constituted persons or things or a force brought to bear on already constituted phenomena. The place of genes as either causal or contributory in these accounts is, then, ambiguous.

The discussions of evidence in the genetic reviews frequently canvass important caveats and limitations, raising further questions about causation. For example, Agrawal and Lynskey (2008) note the importance of family studies in developing understandings of alcoholism but then concede that '[t]he family design cannot distinguish whether the causes of familial similarity [e.g. alcoholism] are genetic or environmental in nature'. They also discuss five 'important limitations' of adoption studies (that they are uncommon, tend to focus on 'paternal alcoholism',[7] do not study families representative of the general population, cannot control for environmental 'exposures' occurring before adoption and do not take into account that the adoption process itself may be 'pathogenic'). The authors then ignore these limitations when they conclude with the following unequivocal statement: 'adoption studies demonstrate a strong link between the biological parent's substance use and offspring risk for addiction, thus establishing that genetic influences are important etiological factors for addiction' (Agrawal & Lynskey 2008, 1071).

Agrawal and Lynskey provide a final stark example of the 'washing away' of the stabilising work being done in relation to evidence in their discussion of twin studies and 'heritability', which they define as the 'proportion of the total phenotypic variance that can be attributed to genetic factors'. The authors place four 'caveats' on the estimates derived from 'simple' twin studies, all of which have been the subject of broader debate in gene research: such studies assume that the researched twins are exposed to and respond equally to their shared environments (irrespective of gender, a point we noted above), neglect uninherited genetic modifications, assume random (rather than assortative) 'mating' between parents and, most strikingly, do not consider the interaction between gene and environment but treat them separately as 'direct effects' (as the authors themselves concede, '[i]n reality, this is rarely the case'). Following their outline of these caveats, Agrawal and Lynskey (2008, 1072) ask readers to '[keep] these limitations in mind' when considering the 'incredible wealth of information in this area' and urge them to 'refer to the exciting empirical research papers' they cite in the following sections of the review. In short, rather than a request for sober reflection, their plea sounds suspiciously like an invitation to allow excitement to overrule reservations about the strength of evidence.

Related to the particular treatment of evidence and causation in these reviews, and bearing in mind our previous point regarding the washing away of caveats and limitations, the fifth collateral reality we identify in the texts is that of science as progress, as constituting an inevitable march towards truth. Great confidence is displayed by the authors regarding the quality of existing evidence, and in line with this enthusiasm they are relentlessly optimistic about the power of science to reveal the reality of alcohol addiction (see Fraser & Seear 2011 for a related argument about hepatitis C science). Consider the following examples:

> new technologies ... are available, enabling a detailed exploration of the genome function and promising an increase of our knowledge of mechanisms through which genetic variation influence protein level/function and environment interacts with the genome.
>
> (Ducci & Goldman 2008, 1422)

> In this exciting time of gene discovery ... with rapid advances in technology (and reductions in cost), gene discovery efforts are likely to accelerate in the near future. Identification of specific genes conveying increased risks have promise not only for understanding the causes and potential treatment for disease, but also for increasing our understanding of how genetic and environmental risks interact to shape liability to addiction.
>
> (Agrawal & Lynskey 2008, 1077)

In these quotations, new genetic methodologies promise to deliver new knowledge. Other parts of the review acknowledge the severe paucity of existing findings, but even this apparent failure is cause for optimism and celebration:

> Although most of the genetic determinants of alcoholism remain to be discovered there are reasons for optimism. In recent years a technological revolution has occurred... [specific genomes] can now be assessed at a level of detail that was previously inconceivable... these tools promise to increase our understanding of the mechanisms by which genetic variation alters molecular function and predisposes individuals to alcoholism and other diseases.
>
> (Ducci & Goldman 2008, 1423)

> The road to the implication of G [gene] x E [environment] studies in (clinical) practice is still long but, to quote Kaufman and Gelernter...'we are not discouraged by the failure to consistently replicate gene-environmental interactions, rather extremely excited by the potential of new investigative techniques to study risk and resiliency across species'.
>
> (Van der Zwaluw & Engels 2009, 911)

In other words, results so far have been disappointing, but the authors remain extremely excited.

This is not to say that all scientists in the area wholeheartedly agree with efforts to find the genetic basis for alcohol addiction. Attempts to stabilise alcohol addiction as a genetic condition, or the result of interactions between genes and environment, have been criticised from within the same ontological and epistemological paradigm. For example, in a Viewpoint article published in the leading journal *Science*, geneticists Merikangas and Risch (2003, 599) highlight the 'continuing difficulty of identifying genes for complex disorders' such as 'alcohol dependence' in a 'robust, replicable manner' and question the 'cost and potential applications of this work to public health'. While they do not spell out the ontological status they ascribe to complex disorders in general and alcohol dependence in particular, their comments suggest the same epistemological paradigm as those they criticise. Doubts are warranted about the 'reliability and validity of phenotypic characterization for complex diseases', partly because this characterisation is 'based primarily on diagnostic criteria obtained from a clinical interview'. In other words, complex human disorders exist but are difficult to identify and measure. Merikangas and Risch identify a second problem with genetics research: the significant contribution of environmental factors to complex diseases, which suggests that these diseases are 'most amenable to environmental modification'. As a result, 'gene hunting for disorders that appear to be highly amenable to environmental modification, such as type 2 diabetes, AIDS, alcohol dependence, and nicotine dependence, would have lower priority, even though genes may be involved in their etiology'. Merikangas and Risch summarise their position thus:

> We need to study behavioral motivation and effective methods for inducing changes in human behavior before we can even begin to envision genetic counseling for disorders such as nicotine or alcohol dependence. It is also unlikely that knowledge of the genes that may accelerate their consequences will alter this situation. Although these behaviors may have some genetic underpinnings, we are still a long way from identifying them. (2003, 601)

More recently, Kalant (2010), a medical pharmacologist, offered another internal critique of genetic research, although the focus is neurobiology rather than genes per se (see our earlier comment on 'genetics' and 'neuroscience'). He also adopts the ontological position that the pathological 'problem' of 'addiction' – a 'behavioral disorder' – does indeed exist and demonstrates a similar epistemological faith in the power of science to reveal its origins. Present, too, is the now familiar apparently relentless optimism about new scientific developments:

> The past two decades have seen dramatic and rapid progress in the field of neurobiology, resulting from the application of a dazzling array of new techniques... It would be impossible to cover here the whole range of new knowledge arising from such work. (2010, 781)

Kalant (2010, 780) qualifies this enthusiasm, however, arguing that 'in relation to addiction this information is of limited value because almost every cell function appears to be involved' and because 'neurons adapt to "addictive drugs" as they do to all sorts of other functional disturbances'. As a result, such information 'may be of limited help in the development of potential auxiliary agents for treatment of addiction' and a 'reductionist approach' attempting to 'analyse addiction at ever finer levels of structure and function' is 'inherently incapable of explaining what causes these mechanisms to be brought into play in some cases and not others'. In his view, there is 'abundant evidence that psychological, social, economic and specific situational factors play important roles in initiating addiction'. Kalant therefore proposes a more integrative approach to studying the 'complex interaction of drug, user, environment and specific situations':

> This is no longer the terrain of pharmacology or neurobiology or psychology or sociology, but an amalgam of all of them. The challenge for research is to find a conceptual framework that can generate the appropriate methods for investigating such an immensely complex system. (2010, 786)

In Kalant's plea for multidisciplinary research, he echoes the ontological and epistemological position we noted earlier (Edwards 1986; see also Carter & Hall 2010): that addiction to alcohol and other drugs exists – as an 'immensely complex system' – and that diverse (if integrated) approaches are required to better understand and treat this condition.

In addition to the inherent complexity of 'addiction', Kalant focuses on some of the other issues we have addressed above. He raises the question of agency in his assertion that 'addiction is not produced by a drug, but by [compulsive] self-administration of a drug' (2010, 781). His declaration that this is ' "real" addiction' locates compulsion (that is, malign agency) within the drug user, therefore apparently contradicting his call for multidisciplinary research on the complex interactions of drug, user, environment and specific situations. He also addresses the thorny question of causation: previous neurobiological research has revealed the '*mechanisms* of cellular adaptive responses' but a 'mechanism is not the same as a *cause*...the cause is that which calls the mechanism into action and directs it toward the relevant and appropriate response' (Kalant 2010, 782). Later on the same page, he states that '[k]nowledge of these mechanisms can tell us *how* the change is brought about, but not *why*'. Most tellingly, Kalant singles out one of neurobiology's central tropes for criticism, providing a different critique from that we offered in Chapter 1:

> [T]he whole concept of the dopaminergic mesolimbic and mesocortical pathways as a 'reward system' must be regarded as a convenient label rather than a literal fact, and it provides no insight into the reasons why some drug users become addicted while the great majority of users, in whom the drugs also stimulate dopamine release in the nucleus accumbens, never pass from use to compulsive use. (2010, 784)

In summary, genetic research occupies the space identified but left unaddressed by work on the alcohol dependence syndrome, locating addiction in the narrowly biological brain and body. It constitutes alcohol addiction as an anterior entity existing independently of the terms used to define it, encompasses virtually all alcohol use in its definition of the 'problem' of alcohol, simplifies 'environment' to allow its measurement and linkage to specific genes, downplays the caveats associated with genetic evidence and trusts science to eventually uncover the reality of alcohol addiction. While there are continuities with the collateral realities enacted in previous work on alcohol dependence, genetic approaches move alcohol dependence more explicitly into a biomedical space. Alongside these attempts to stabilise alcohol addiction as genetic, attempts to re-assemble alcohol addiction as a 'disorder' emerged in the proposed revisions to the *DSM-5*. In the next section, we turn to these attempts because they again highlight how a concept taken by many to be stable and self-evident is, in expert circles, highly volatile, unstable and ambiguous: subjected over and again to criticism, revision and re-definition.

A new object: 'Alcohol use disorder'

As we noted in Chapter 1, over the last decade the American Psychiatric Association (APA) examined and revised the criteria used in the *DSM-IV* to diagnose and classify mental disorders. This process of examination and revision culminated in the release of the *DSM-5* in May 2013. In the discussions that took place during the examination and revision process, addiction became the subject of intense scholarly debate.[8] This debate focused on the APA's proposal to replace the categories of 'substance dependence' and 'substance abuse' with 'substance use disorder'. As we also noted in Chapter 1, this change, along with others proposed in the revision, was justified on several grounds: continuity, clarity and conciseness; new research evidence; ease of use for clinicians and greater flexibility with regard to diverse patient and client groups. In this section, we examine in detail a specific instance of this debate in order to explore its wider significance for changing definitions of addiction and the collateral realities being enacted in the process of stabilising it. It involves an exchange published in 2012 in the *Journal of Studies on Alcohol and Drugs*. This consisted of a letter written by Griffith Edwards (2012 – at the time of writing, the most downloaded article in the journal for that year), in which he argues against the proposed changes to the *DSM-IV*, and responses to his letter from three members of the

APA's Substance-Related Disorders Work Group: Charles O'Brien (2012), a psychiatrist and chair of the work group; Deborah Hasin (2012), a psychiatric epidemiologist; and Marc Schuckit (2012), a psychiatrist and the editor of the journal. We do not analyse O'Brien's response here as he refers exclusively to the use of opiates in his discussion of 'dependence' and 'addiction' (but see Keane et al. 2011).

We argue that the proposal to adopt the term 'alcohol use disorder' in the *DSM-5* attempted to stabilise a new pathological object, doing so using some now familiar strategies:

- the continuing conceptualisation of alcohol addiction as an anterior object;
- the pathologisation of an ever wider range of drinking practices;
- the marshalling of epidemiological evidence to support the move to 'disorder' despite its methodological and conceptual limitations;
- the simplifying of environment and the 'social'; and
- the valorisation of biomedical research as the paramount form of scientific explanation.

Although these strategies are similar to those explored in previous sections, they emerge in a different institutional context and for different ends – as a response to calls for improved diagnostic measures. The general point is that, regardless of the type of account being offered (psychiatric, genetic, epidemiological), the overall intention remains the same: to simplify and stabilise alcohol addiction. As we saw in the responses to the claims made in genetic research on alcohol addiction, the attempt to stabilise 'disorder' as a new object in the *DSM-5* was met with considerable opposition. This time it came from those wedded to the original formulation of alcohol dependence and its conceptual distinction from other forms of drinking.

Edwards (2012) opens his letter with an historical outline of ideas about addiction from the early 1800s to the present. This account evokes the collateral reality seen in previous sections: that of a stable, constant and pathological anterior 'syndrome', 'a recognizable clinical entity', around which diverse terminology – addiction, inebriety and alcoholism – has historically gathered. After detailing previous debates about the introduction of the term 'dependence', the bi-axial formulation of 'dependence' and 'problems', and the institutional processes underlying the development of the *DSM* and the WHO's *International Classification of Diseases*, Edwards focuses specifically on two of the proposed changes to the conceptualisation of alcohol (and other drug) dependence in the *DSM-5*. The two proposed changes were that the term 'dependence' should be replaced by 'disorder' and that the 'abuse' category should be removed. First, Edwards (2012, 700) argues that 'although a number of debatable points are being made, no convincing case, either clinical or scientific, is established for the proposed change in nomenclature [from "dependence" to "disorder"]'. In his view, 'the impression is given of a field in disarray' (Edwards 2012, 701). Second, Edwards criticises the removal of the 'abuse' category, and the consequent loss of the '"problems" dimension', from the *DSM-5*. He makes this case on two grounds: (1) that the removal of the category of 'abuse' ignores clinical, epidemiological and anthropological evidence that 'suggests that people can develop destructive and disruptive drinking behavior without clinical symptoms of dependence', and (2) that it relies on a specific interpretation of recent US drinking surveys in order to argue that there is 'no distinct entity of dependence that is discontinuous with nondependent drinking problems' (Edwards 2012, 701). He argues that the 'possibility exists... that the questions used in [this] type of research are technically insufficient to discriminate troubled drinking without dependence from the dependence syndrome' (2012, 701).

Edwards enacts three related collateral realities in these claims. First, in citing clinical, epidemiological and anthropological evidence,[9] he again poses drinking as best understood through a multidisciplinary lens, but only in so far as all contributing disciplines proceed on the assumption that the 'clinical symptoms of dependence' can be separated from other forms of drinking. In other words, they must accept a second collateral reality: dependence as an identifiable, stable and distinct syndrome. Third, he critiques the epidemiological research used to support the change to 'disorder'. But his epistemological critique is a careful one for he also relies on the collateral reality of epidemiological evidence to make his first point. Rather than questioning the epidemiological enterprise as a whole, its tendency to rely upon highly reductive questions, his critique is specific: the *particular* questions used in the cited US surveys cannot identify and separate the dependence syndrome from 'troubled drinking without dependence'. By removing the categories of 'dependence' and 'abuse' and replacing them with 'disorder', the two-dimensional view of alcohol-related problems, so fundamental to his original formulation of the alcohol dependence syndrome, to earlier versions of the *DSM* and to public health approaches to drinking (see, for example, Babor et al. 2001, 2010), has been collapsed into a unidimensional view.

What other collateral realities are being performed in the merging of 'alcohol dependence' and 'alcohol abuse' and replacement with 'alcohol use disorder'? As Edwards notes, until the 1960s, 'alcoholism' served as an umbrella term for drinking problems. In the late 1970s, following the publication of Edwards and Gross (1976) and associated research, 'alcoholism' was replaced by a bi-axial formulation – 'alcohol dependence' and 'alcohol-related problems' – with the former characterised by the seven criteria outlined by Edwards and Gross and the latter referring to more general problems including those of an acute kind. With the proposing and adoption of the term 'alcohol use disorder' in the *DSM-5*, we see a return to an umbrella term that collapses the bi-axial formulation. This return to a unidimensional model seems to repeat history. Jellinek's (1960) five subtypes of 'alcoholism' covered a wide range of drinking patterns, including the kind of drinking that later became understood as 'dependence' – characterised by impaired control, tolerance and withdrawal – as well as the form of drinking that is now commonly described as binge drinking. The term 'alcohol use disorder' performs a similarly collapsing function: it brings under the same umbrella term very different forms of drinking – from the occasional binge drinking of young adults through to the daily heavy drinking of the stereotypically 'dependent' drinker. It seems drinking alcohol is a disorder no matter what form it takes. This terminological revision extends the pathology, compulsion and stigmatisation associated with dependence to many different forms of drinking.

The first response to Edwards's letter is from Deborah Hasin (2012), a psychiatric epidemiologist and member of the APA's Substance-Related Disorders Work Group, who focuses on his objection to the proposed removal of the 'abuse' category in the *DSM-5*. She accepts the 'conceptual distinction' between 'the dependence process and its consequences' and acknowledges that the 'conceptual formulations of Griffith Edwards's *dependence syndrome* (Edwards & Gross 1976) have had an enormous influence on the measurement of substance use disorders' (Hasin 2012, 702). But she then addresses 'the concern about combining abuse and dependence, thereby *eliminating* the abuse category [emphasis added]'. Notwithstanding Hasin's phrasing, her view is that 'abuse' and 'dependence' have not been combined in the *DSM-5*; rather, 'abuse' has been 'eliminated', presumably to be absorbed within the category of 'dependence', which has then been renamed 'disorder'. Here problems (or, for Hasin, 'consequences') such as violence or accidents associated with what we might call 'acute' consumption (such as binge drinking amongst young people) have been conceptually aligned with problems theorised to arise from a pathological psychobiological core. With 'abuse' eliminated, the characteristics of 'dependence' are left intact, relabelled as 'disorder' and applied to all drinking problems. The political implications of this move are profound: whereas the concept of dependence posited a theory of drinking problems based on social learning and biology, 'disorder' is solely an assessment of conduct (a negative and stigmatising one) that can be applied to a wider range of drinking practices and those engaging in them.

Hasin also enacts a very simple reality of the social. She agrees that Edwards's original description 'conceptually differentiated the dependence syndrome from other substance-related physical, mental, and social disabilities in a bi-axial formulation' (Hasin 2012, 702). Here, 'social disabilities' are produced as characteristics of individual subjects rather than the emergent outcome of specific assemblages – for example, violence as an outcome of the assemblage of alcohol, bodies, emotions, forms of masculinity and drinking spaces (Jayne et al. 2010). Her response also describes thoroughly social and cultural phenomena – such as interpersonal problems or the neglect of social roles and obligations – as 'symptoms' as in 'the relationship between abuse and dependence symptoms'.

Like Edwards, Hasin draws on epidemiological research to make her case. She cites US and other surveys that show continuity rather than discontinuity between dependence and abuse: in other words, as dependence becomes more severe, so too do abuse 'indicators'. For this reason, she argues that 'a one-factor model that incorporated both dependence and abuse criteria... fit the data better than a two-factor model that differentiated between these two types of criteria' (Hasin 2012, 702). In using this epidemiological evidence, she acknowledges the criticisms of Edwards (2012) and others (for example, Caetano & Babor 2006) that the measures used in these surveys are problematic and also details some of the limitations of the epidemiology on which her argument relies: that it requires instruments that are easy to administer and therefore struggles to capture the complexity of 'real-world issues'; that the severity of some of the alcohol use disorder diagnostic criteria is greater in treatment samples than in surveys of the general population; and that the relationship between abuse and dependence criteria might differ between general population and clinical samples. Despite these significant limitations, and her stated acceptance of the conceptual difference between alcohol dependence and alcohol abuse, she concludes that in the face of the 'overwhelming abundance of evidence in favor of combining the abuse and dependence criteria, I found I no longer had grounds to hold to my position' (Hasin 2012, 703). Despite her reliance on epidemiological evidence, Hasin further complicates and undermines its status when she closes her response by holding out hope for the discovery of 'indicators of the dependence syndrome process at a more endophenotypic level' – in other words, that genetic research will ultimately deliver the truth about addiction. Here, again, we see enacted the collateral reality of science, especially biomedical science, as capable of revealing the ultimate truth about addiction.

The second response to Edwards's letter is from Marc Schuckit (2012), a psychiatrist, editor of the journal in which the exchange appears and member of the APA's Substance-Related Disorders Work Group. First, like Hasin, he invokes two by now familiar collateral realities – that epidemiological evidence warrants the adoption of 'disorder' and that biomedicine (in the form of gene science) is best placed to identify its ontologically anterior 'essence' – dependence – and to provide definitive answers to the problems of diagnosis. As he puts it, 'If... sensitive, specific, reliable, and valid biological criteria could be found, there might be less room for disagreement regarding the best way to diagnose [substance-related] disorders' (Schuckit 2012, 521). Because we currently lack such criteria, he argues, 'the essence of SUDs [substance use disorders] has not yet been clearly identified'. Like Edwards (1986) and Li et al. (2007), Schuckit also invokes multidisciplinarity:

> If they approach [the elephant] from the front, they might accurately perceive a large, soft protuberance and long eyelashes, but the view from behind could be quite different... Both views are correct, but neither gives the entire picture. Similarly, I think we have a decent feel for the SUDs we study and treat, but we don't yet fully understand the entire beast. (2012, 521)

The addiction-as-elephant metaphor is worth considering in some detail here. In another article canvassing some of the same issues covered by Schuckit, Li et al. also describe alcohol addiction as an elephant:[10]

> [I]t [the evolution of views on 'alcohol use and its problems' and conceptual differences in the definition of these problems] is reminiscent of the old saw about blind-folded observers defining what an elephant is by only the portion that they can feel. To begin to see the 'whole animal', it is first useful to understand the differences between definition of a disease and its diagnosis. (2007, 1523)

One could hardly hope for clearer examples of what STS theorist Annemarie Mol calls 'perspectivalism' or the gathering of diverse experts around an object enacted as anterior to observation:

> Perspectivalism broke away from a monopolistic version of truth. But it didn't multiply *reality*. It multiplied the eyes of the beholders... While in the centre the object of the many gazes and glances remains singular, intangible, untouched. (1999, 75–76)

The SUD elephant – the 'entire beast' or the 'whole animal' – exists prior to and independent of the various perspectives adopted by its observers. Like Hasin, Schuckit cites epidemiological studies in support of dropping the 'abuse' category from the *DSM-5* but, oddly, claims that the 'proposed *DSM-5* approach to SUDs allows researchers and clinicians to continue to pay attention to the abuse criteria that have been part of the DSM since 1987'. In Schuckit's scheme, the abuse criteria remain, but they now go to diagnosing a 'disorder' which, in turn, is treated as equivalent to 'dependence' but without recognition of the conceptual differences between alcohol dependence as a compulsive condition and forms of drinking problems seen to arise from different origins and understood from different perspectives.

What all of this does is apply dependence (now called disorder) to a wider population, in what we referred to in Chapter 1 as 'diagnostic bracket creep'. This is precisely the criticism made by prominent alcohol policy researchers quoted in an article that appeared in *The New York Times* – 'Addiction diagnoses may rise under guideline changes' (Urbina 2012, accessed on 11 August 2013, www.nytimes.com/2012/05/12/us/dsm-revisions-may-sharply-increase-addiction-diagnoses.html?pagewanted=all&_r=0). In support of its claim the article refers to an Australian study (Mewton et al. 2011) which shows that the new *DSM-5* criteria would result in a 61% increase in the diagnosis of an alcohol use disorder compared to the *DSM-IV* criteria. The article also quotes Thomas Babor, Associate Editor-in-Chief of *Addiction* and lead author of influential alcohol policy textbook *Alcohol: No Ordinary Commodity* (Babor et al. 2010): 'The chances of getting a diagnosis [of addiction] are going to be much greater, and this will artificially inflate the statistics considerably... These sorts of diagnoses could be a real embarrassment.' Babor's fear is that such inflation could lead to scarce funds being misdirected to those with only 'mild problem[s]' (Urbina 2012).

Schuckit refers to the *New York Times* article and the concerns expressed in it in a journal press release announcing the publication of the exchange between Edwards, Hasin, O'Brien and Schuckit: 'It was unfortunate that *The New York Times* article had some major inaccuracies.' He does not identify the inaccuracies (much less refute them) and says that a comparison of the *DSM-IV* and *DSM-5* schemes 'found that the number of people diagnosed did not change much across the two'. The press release contains no figures to support this statement.

In summary, the proposed changes to the *DSM-5,* which Edwards opposed and Hasin and Schuckit (as well as by other researchers such as Li et al.) advocate, constitute alcohol addiction and its collateral realities in several ways. They continue to conceptualise alcohol addiction as an anterior object, pathologise an ever wider range of drinking practices, marshal epidemiological evidence to support the move to 'disorder' despite its acknowledged methodological and conceptual limitations, simplify environment and valorise biomedical research as the ultimate form of scientific explanation. Here, addiction is extended and re-made to address calls for improved diagnostic instruments.

Conclusion

In this chapter we analysed changing definitions and collateral realities of alcohol addiction. We focused in particular on several key debates that have constituted and reconstituted alcohol addiction, arguing that the concept is, in expert circles, highly volatile, ambiguous and slippery, always open to redefinition, even as the condition it purports to denote is repeatedly constituted as anterior and pathological. Unlike the vigorous stabilising of methamphetamine addiction, which, by comparison, appears relatively settled and coherent, we see new definitions, critiques and debates about alcohol addiction emerging over time.

In our discussion of Robin Room's research we argued that sociological accounts developed a binary analytical framework in which 'alcoholism', 'alcohol addiction' and 'alcohol dependence' are socially constructed or framed but their material realities (of biology and pharmacology) pre-exist this construction or framing, remaining ontologically separate from it. Psychiatric research constituting and stabilising the 'alcohol dependence syndrome' enacted several collateral realities: clinical knowledge and the need to treat problem drinkers demand new ways of thinking about alcoholism, dependence constitutes a definite 'syndrome' that can be treated despite its description remaining 'provisional', dependence is an ontologically anterior 'pathological process' best understood through multidisciplinary research, and (narrowly conceived) environments are external to the 'psychobiological core' of dependence. Genetic research on alcohol also enacted several collateral realities (many of which echo or mesh with those relied upon in the preceding formulation): alcohol addiction is an ontologically anterior entity, the 'problem' of alcohol encompasses virtually all alcohol use, the 'environment' must be simplified in order to allow its measurement and linkage to specific genes, the limitations of genetic evidence can be ignored, and science will eventually uncover the reality of alcohol addiction. Finally, we showed how the proposal to adopt the term 'alcohol use disorder' in the *DSM-5* enacted a further set of collateral realities (again showing some overlap with those it aimed to supersede or replace): alcohol addiction again as an anterior object, the pathology of an ever wider range of drinking practices, epidemiological evidence as warranting the move to 'disorder' despite its methodological and conceptual limitations, the environment and the 'social' as comprising a narrow range of elements, and biomedical research as the paramount means of uncovering the truth of alcohol dependence.

In tracking the collateral realities being constituted in the different debates on alcohol addiction, as well as those relating to methamphetamine addiction explored in previous chapters, three further observations can be made. First, there is a good deal of overlap in the collateral realities being used to stabilise very different addiction objects: for example, addiction is an anterior pathological process or entity, limitations in evidence can be ignored, simplified conceptualisations of environment are adequate and scientific research (especially biomedical research) will eventually provide definitive answers to key questions. These overlaps suggests that the different positions taken in these debates – addiction as psychological, addiction as a brain disease, addiction as psychobiological, addiction as genetic, addiction as disorder – share the same ontological foundations and that developing new ways of thinking about addiction requires more fundamental revision than is possible within the parameters of these debates. The second observation we make about the collateral realities being constituted in debates on alcohol and methamphetamine addiction also concerns their similarity. If, as we argue, addiction is an assemblage, made and remade in different ways in discourse but stabilised through the enactment of similar collateral realities, then these enactments might also be understood as habits: that is, as regular or settled tendencies or practices – relating to ontology, epistemology, pathology and agency – that are hard to forsake and which emerge repeatedly in different research, policy and public accounts of addiction. Finally, how are we to understand a process in which different objects of addiction are being stabilised through the enactment of overlapping collateral realities? Law (2011, 165) argues that different objects are enacted at different moments according to different needs and that 'such multiplicity is a necessary condition for institutional survival'. Each of the attempts to stabilise alcohol use and addiction does not hold, or does not hold for long, always threatening to implode under attack from new research and medical technology, various policy imperatives such as increasing concern over binge drinking amongst young people and the public health burden of drinking, and calls for improved diagnostic instruments. Perhaps, over time, we will witness with methamphetamine and obesity the same cycle of definition, critique and debate, particularly if overeating continues to draw attention as yet another form of addiction.

In Chapter 3, we showed how individuals experienced in methamphetamine consumption frequently articulated ideas about the drug, its consumers and addiction in terms that reproduced and sometimes challenged those found in research and policy discourse. As the collateral realities of methamphetamine addiction emerged as relatively stable, so too did methamphetamine addiction itself. In the next chapter, we analyse interviews on alcohol use and its effects conducted with young people – one of the key population groups of most concern in alcohol policy – examining how closely some of the collateral realities most persistently enacted across these different expert debates resemble those young people enact in their accounts of drinking.

5
Assembling Alcohol Problems: Young People and Drinking

In the previous chapter we examined in detail the debates that have constituted and re-constituted alcohol addiction or 'dependence' since 1976, arguing that a concept many take to be stable and self-evident is, in expert circles, highly volatile: subjected over and over to criticism and revision. This instability and controversy mark alcohol addiction out from the methamphetamine addiction found in Chapters 2 and 3 to be so vigorously subject to stabilisation. In tracking methamphetamine addiction concepts across research, policy and consumer or public settings, we found that individual methamphetamine consumers frequently (although not always) articulated ideas about the drug, about those who consume it and why, and about the addiction with which it is associated, in terms highly consonant with research and policy discourse. As these ideas – that is, the collateral realities enacted in the production of methamphetamine addiction – emerge as relatively stable, so too does methamphetamine addiction itself.

In this chapter we conduct a process of comparison similar to that undertaken in Chapters 2 and 3. In this case, our focus is on the relationship between research and public understandings of alcohol addiction rather than of methamphetamine addiction. We undertake this comparison using interviews conducted with young drinkers (instead of methamphetamine consumers), assessing the connections and divergences between the articulations of alcohol addiction found in research discussed in Chapter 4 and public ones. Perhaps unsurprisingly, given the instability of alcohol dependence in the research and the variable role of drinking in everyday life, young people talk about alcohol and its effects in very different ways. Cause and effect, the role of environment, the nature of the phenomenon of alcohol addiction – all these central issues are treated more ambivalently than is found in discussions of methamphetamine. As we argued in Chapter 4, the core object of alcohol addiction proves slippery and difficult to stabilise. Little distinction is made in the interviews we conducted between 'alcohol problems' in general and addiction in particular, and although some signifiers of problematic consumption are readily cited, these are oftentimes subsumed under broader statements about assessing the problem in context. Perhaps ironically, perhaps fittingly, we find many of our participants demur when asked about how alcohol addiction can be identified, reminding us that in practice 'it depends'.

One way of reading these interview accounts to grasp the contingency articulated within them is to revisit the notion of the assemblage on which John Law's work is partly based (following Latour). Such accounts, we might say, see alcohol dependence much as the authors of this book do – made in practice, only possible in the confluence of complex and emergent phenomena, difficult to stabilise in the multiplicity of their ontological constituents. This, as we will show, would be partly right. At the same time that alcohol addiction is made in such ontologically multiple ways, however, many statements also treat it as ontologically singular: self-evident and anterior to discourses of addiction. Alcohol addiction has, it seems, many partial enactments, sometimes taken for granted, sometimes subjected to scepticism and critique. As Law explains in his discussion of ontological politics and the production of collateral realities, 'different realities are enacted at different moments according to different needs'.

In this chapter we begin by looking briefly at the sociological literature on drinking over the last decade. This literature has followed shifts in expert discourse on alcohol by increasingly focusing on youth and binge or heavy sessional drinking and away from the traditional figure of the alcoholic as an older, heavy daily consumer. In discussing this literature, we consider (much as we did with Robin Room's work in the previous chapter) the ways in which it understands the ontology of drinking, using a recent article to draw out the relevance of our theoretical framework (Law's mobilisation of concepts of the assemblage and collateral realities) for better conceptualising and understanding drinking. Following this, we turn to 30 interviews conducted with young people in Melbourne, Australia, to examine the ways in which they understand drinking, alcohol problems and alcohol addiction. We ask, how closely do young people's articulations of alcohol and drinking relate to those found in the research discussed in the previous chapter? Are the realities being stabilised in the research also being stabilised in youth public discourse? How readily are the collateral realities used to achieve the (somewhat transitory or imperfect) stabilities found in the expert debates enacted in young people's articulations of alcohol and addiction? As with the other two sections in this book (on the methamphetamine 'crisis', and the rise of 'food addiction' via the neuroscience of overweight and obesity) our aim is to explore the trajectories of meaning and practice that emerge for addiction in its mutual constitution with specific substances and specific public health target groups. More generally, we also aim to examine the fate of addiction as it operates across these three very different material-discursive contexts (methamphetamine, alcohol and food). After all, if (as we observed in the book's Introduction) the minimum unit of reality is the assemblage, then addiction is an assemblage of material and non-material phenomena, its reality held stable via the enactment of particular collateral realities. These must be identified and examined if any thorough comprehension of addiction and its changing shape can be achieved.

Youth drinking: Social science and its metaphors

Concern about the growth in alcohol consumption among young people has appeared in the social science literature since the late 1990s (Balding 1997; Socialstyrelsen 1997; Pedersen & Skrondal 1998). Researchers have sought to define, explain and evaluate this growth, identifying, for example, factors linked to specific drinking patterns (Kloep et al. 2001; Measham & Brain 2005; Lindsay 2009; Fry 2010; Heimisdottir et al. 2010), and considering the relative importance of generational norms versus national norms in shaping patterns of consumption (Järvinen & Room 2007). Some discussion has even been had over the direction of drinking trends depending upon the dates compared (Measham 2008). As Measham puts it in her 2007 article on youth drinking in the United Kingdom since 2000:

> Depending on one's historical perspective, alcohol consumption can be increasing, decreasing, or stable. For example, a cut-off point of the 1950s would suggest that alcohol consumption has increased steadily for the last 50 years or so. However, a cut-off point back in the nineteenth century would suggest that the increases since the 1950s are only a return to pre-twentieth century levels following a decline in consumption in the first half of the twentieth century with the impact of two world wars and their aftermath. (2007, 208)

Measham points out that the debates about alcohol consumption played out in the media and in academic contexts relate to more general concerns about the 'problems' of youth, working-class leisure and deviance. The problem of excessive drinking is, according to this view, an effect of broader social discourses which are themselves highly political. These are important observations that set questions about drinking in a wider context than public health responses tend to recognise. Measham's aim in the article is to bring together survey and interview data across a range of studies to describe and assess emerging changes in drinking patterns among youth. She argues that drinking patterns are polarising, with some young people embracing drinking to excess ('determined drunkenness') and the social and economic frameworks that support it, while others have turned to abstinence as a reaction to this trend.

Measham's article covers a great deal of ground, taking in commercial forces, laws about public consumption of alcohol and public disorder, and the privatisation of public space, in its assessment of the factors contributing to youth drinking and to the specific shape it has taken over time (her view is that rates have levelled off since 2000). In doing so, she does not theorise her approach in any explicit way. For this reason, the way in which she conceives the object of her analysis – youth drinking – remains somewhat unclear. On the one hand, her observations about the politics behind particular problematisations of youth drinking, and her investigation of factors that contribute to drinking patterns at different times and in different places, suggest an approach in keeping with our own in this book, one where the object of analysis is conceived as an assemblage rather than a stable bounded object anterior to its description. On the other hand, the absence of any overt consideration of such theoretical issues, and the conclusion's observations about the importance of considering the effect of 'context' on drinking habits, would seem to reaffirm drinking as a bounded object against which a context can be defined. Why should a distinction of this kind matter for our study of alcohol and its relationship with discourses of addiction? Why should it matter for understandings of youth drinking practices? A brief examination of one of the most innovative research articles to emerge from the recent sociological engagement with youth drinking helps to clarify this. Then we turn to our empirical material and our broader task: an examination of the relationship between research debate about alcohol and addiction and the articulations found among the target audience of public health translations of these debates into health messages.

In 2012 Brown and Gregg published an article on young Australian and UK women's drinking patterns and use of Facebook. The article distinguishes itself by looking closely at two contemporary trends at once, paying a similar level of attention to both. Arguing that drug education pedagogy does not take into account the pleasure young women find in intoxication and the online narratives they produce about it, the article criticises the emphasis in drug education on heavily gendered notions of sexual vulnerability and regret. Not only are young women invited to consider themselves permanently at risk of loss of control and agency in their social experiences of drinking, they are also expected to look back on sexual encounters while intoxicated with regret and even shame. Messages of this kind are not, Brown and Gregg point out, directed at young men too. That such normalising, implicitly judgemental and stigmatising messages about female sexuality continue to be promulgated in the name of health is obviously cause for concern in itself. Yet as Brown and Gregg point out, this is not the only problem with the approach. As even a cursory look at young women's Facebook pages indicates, intoxication and the various transgressions understood to accompany it belong to a much bigger set of practices and concerns for young women. In short, they act as the building blocks for important processes of self-making in that they form an important source of material for Facebook entries and for online socialising in general. A night out, we are told, comprises a combination of two key pleasures: intoxication *and* Facebooking. As Brown and Gregg explain:

> The 'peak' of the night out is also routinely documented by the live post or photo update, as mobile devices allow a narrative thread to be maintained for onlookers. One of the amusements for the Facebook audience is in discerning the moment of intoxication, either during or after the event. Telltale signs are when words which may have been chosen carefully just hours earlier become careless, provocative or even incoherent. (2012, 363)

As the authors go on to argue (2012, 363), 'Facebook and drinking are thus a twinned entertainment, in that the experience of each is mutually enhanced in combination.'

Brown and Gregg make a very important argument here in linking intoxication and social networking technology. Yet their metaphorical characterisation of the two as 'twinned' raises its own questions: in particular, it leaves undertheorised the connections between the phenomena. The relationship between intoxication and social networking technologies is construed, we would argue, only very sketchily in the metaphor of the twin. Indeed, we can find several ambiguities implicit in the idea, especially if we analyse it perhaps more literally than intended – after all, such unintended meanings cannot be ignored in assessing the effects of metaphors (see Keane 2002; Fraser & valentine 2008). As we have argued elsewhere, drawing on the work of Derrida (Fraser & valentine 2008, 41), 'worn-out' metaphors may be 'no longer evident to speakers or listeners, appearing instead as literal language. [Yet] these worn-out metaphors nevertheless help shape the trajectory of our thinking'. This is why – and how – such metaphors matter. To unpack this twin metaphor a little with the help of an equally metaphorical discourse, biology, there are two types of twins: identical and fraternal. The former develop from one fertilised egg that separates into two identical parts, and share the same genes. The latter develop from two separately fertilised eggs and are like siblings in their genetic relationship. Are intoxication and Facebook, then, derived from a single shared source, or have they developed alongside each other from different but related materials? Are they, as foetuses are normally so problematically understood, gestated in a particular 'environment', and if so, what has this environment contributed to their shape and character? Are they thought to have intrinsic, permanent similarities, and a special affinity? Of course, Brown and Gregg do not intend for their use of the word 'twinned' to denote such specificities, but by looking closely at its implications we can see the need for a term that more precisely describes the relationship between the two.

In keeping with the overall approach we take in this book, which understands reality as made in practice, as multiple, and as constituted from unstable, network-like phenomena rather than stable bounded objects, we consider the notion of the assemblage useful here. As Law explains in his chapter on collateral realities (2011, 157):

> Practices then, *are* assemblages of relations. Those assemblages *do* realities. Realities, including the incidental collateral realities, *are inseparable from the patterning juxtapositions of practices.*

As with the question about context that arises in response to other accounts of youth drinking (such as Measham's) that attempt to integrate factors beyond the substance itself into accounts of drinking, the idea of twinning leads to important ontological questions about the nature of reality, the making of objects and other phenomena, and the way in which such phenomena impact on each other. When Brown and Gregg (2012, 364) conclude that '[t]he pedagogy of regret underpinning binge drinking campaigns targeted at youth underestimates the cultural dynamics of leisure practices, including the longer "drunken narrative" ', they remind us that at least three elements are at stake in efforts to protect young women's health and well-being: alcohol consumption, social networking and pedagogical strategy. If these three elements are seen conventionally as essentially independent but fleetingly connected, the ways in which they constitute each other, and can therefore act to reconstitute each other in new ways, is lost. So our point here is not to say, as do Brown and Gregg (2012, 364), that Facebooking extends the pleasures of binge drinking – that it forms part of the 'wider dimensions *accompanying* young people's drinking *habits* [emphasis added]'. Instead we argue that such technological practices help *make* drinking practices, that the relationship is much more interdependent than that of accompaniment, and that habit, whatever it is when it comes to alcohol consumption, is only made possible by the co-production of objects, phenomena and practices. This, indeed, is what habit is: it is another word for reality – something held together only by enactment and reenactment, and by the enactment and reenactment of collateral realities. Entailed in this idea of reality as habit is, of course, that of the assemblage. This is the fundamental ontological unit with which we work in this book, and which describes each and every phenomenon with which we engage. So, in working with Brown and Gregg's valuable study, we might propose that young women's drinking is an assemblage constituted in relation to other assemblages such as available feminine sexualities, broader drinking practices, the substance of alcohol and its presence in variously constituted beverages, and contemporary social networking technologies.

Of course, re-reading the research of others with new theoretical tools is hardly empirically conclusive. Doing so can raise questions, offer hints and suggest possible pathways, but it leaves many questions unanswered, partly because it relies on very limited access to the data on which the published research was based. In the remainder of this chapter we therefore go further, analysing interviews collected for our own work with young people in Melbourne, Australia, and using the theoretical tools described here to produce a different account of youth drinking and meaning-making around alcohol consumption and addiction. In the process we consider the points of similarity, if any, with the research discourse on alcohol problems and addiction discussed in Chapter 4. Given the instability and multiplicity of these research discourses, it is not surprising that we find multiplicity and contradiction in public articulations as well. As we will see, however, three complexly related trends are also evident in the interviews. First, we find a significant degree of *unanimity* on key identifiers of alcohol problems; second, we find a significant *overlap* in the markers of alcohol problems and alcohol addiction; and third, we find, alongside this overlap and unanimity, a noticeable *sensitivity to oversimplification* and a resistance to unidimensional explanations for alcohol problems in general or addiction in particular. It is this last aspect of the data we pay especial attention to in concluding this chapter. As with public accounts of methamphetamine use and, as we will later see, overeating and obesity, the emphasis many place on the complexity and multiplicity of factors at play in the development and persistence of problems to do with consumption demands attention and theorisation. Perhaps for a range of reasons, these interviews differ markedly from research discourse which, especially in relation to questions of the 'environment' in which addiction or problematic use is identified, tends to pursue a high degree of simplification and stabilisation.

It 'depends': Young people make alcohol addiction

In this chapter we focus on two aspects of the interviews we conducted with young people (for details of data collection and analysis, please see the Appendix). These are the statements made in response to two topic areas raised: (1) what is 'problem drinking', or 'a problem with alcohol' and how can it be identified, and (2) what is addiction and how does it relate, if at all, to alcohol consumption. Perhaps the most obvious finding in analysing responses to these two areas is the significant amount of overlap between them for some participants. Some made little, if any, useful distinction between problem drinking and alcohol addiction. In this respect these accounts mirror the instability found in expert discourse surrounding the question of whether a differentiated taxonomy of pathology is viable or desirable. Are 'drinking problems' and addiction – or 'alcohol dependence' – sensibly distinguished? This picture is by no means clear. Parvani (a 24-year-old woman), for example, cites the following identifying features of a person she knows with an 'alcohol problem':

> [he] would prefer to drink every single day and probably like seven, eight drinks every single day of the week…

Here Parvani's watchwords are volume and frequency. These are then connected to social relationships in Parvani's account:

> And the kids aren't too happy with their father.

When asked a more specific question about alcohol *addiction*, Parvani cites the same features: volume and frequency of consumption, confirming that, yes,

> Definitely, I think anyone who's drinking every single day and having like seven, eight glasses of scotch... if someone's not leaving it, then it's addiction.

Parvani's comments suggest at least that alcohol addiction might count as a subset of alcohol problems. However, when other participants are asked to spell out the features of 'alcohol addiction', these cover, almost exhaustively, the same territory as the broader category of problem drinking. Polly (a 23-year-old woman), for instance, frames the issues this way:

> Oh I think it's [drinking] definitely an addiction. I think that anything can become an addiction if it makes someone feel less connected or better. Yeah... I think that you can also become addicted to just binge drinking on the weekends, you know. You might not touch a drink during the week but then, I think for some people, if they have a drink they can't stop so one drink leads to you know twenty.

For Polly, occasional heavy drinking and daily heavy drinking both qualify as addiction. Indeed, addiction is a possibility wherever drinking allows the individual in question to feel 'less connected' (perhaps to problems) or 'better'.

To sum up, the young people we interviewed often cite the same defining features for alcohol problems and for alcohol addiction. These are where drinking

- is excessive in volume,
- is excessive in frequency,
- harms relationships,
- is experienced as a psychological need or operates as a crutch,
- is experienced as a physical need or dependence,

- harms health,
- occurs alone,
- is marked by an absence of control,
- is misrecognised as a solution to worries and other problems,
- disrupts other aspects of life and relationships,
- is required to enable socialising,
- is required every day to feel 'normal',
- is used as an escape from reality or to numb feelings,
- is the only source of pleasure or is essential for feelings of pleasure, such as where a meal is unsatisfying without alcohol, and
- is excessively costly, wasting money.

Clearly, there are many ways in which drinking can register as a problem, and many ways in which this problem is indistinguishable from addiction. In this respect, and in their echoes of the diagnostic criteria described in the previous chapter, the interviews suggest that public accounts of alcohol addiction share something with the controversies in research discourse on alcohol. Should an idea of alcohol addiction or dependence exist alone or should it be subsumed under, and therefore lend weight to, an expansionist category of alcohol consumption that, as we have argued, seeks to gather together almost all drinking under the rubric of the 'problem'? These are questions our interview participants cannot, of course, answer, not least because as a whole, and despite some evident readiness to cite signs of problem drinking, they actually show little interest overall in constructing narrow or universal definitions of healthy and unhealthy drinking beyond some simple statements about individual cases or very specific circumstances. Indeed, a number of participants stated, when asked, that they did not know anyone with a drinking problem.

More specifically, many participants were often hesitant to ascribe problem status or addiction to drinking without attaching many conditions and caveats. Yes, volume and frequency are important, but these matter only in the context of social relationships, work, other attributes of the individual in question and so on. For example, some kinds of drinking thought to hint at a problem or an addiction in an older person are often explained in young people as merely part and parcel of socialising and everyday life. Leila (18), for instance, explained heavy drinking among other young people of her acquaintance in this way:

> No, even my friends drink a lot but they will, they will wake up tomorrow and just feel uncomfortable and that's it, nothing. I think it's not a problem right?

Ling, too, says heavy, or 'binge' drinking is unproblematic. In her view, it is just part of going out. She sees signs of a drinking problem or addiction elsewhere, such as in the practice of drinking alone, or when drinking falls out of a delicate balance with other activities, taking precedence over them instead of enhancing them:

> LING: I don't know anyone who has [a drinking problem] – but it's ... like most people go out to drink, they just usually binge ... so no one that I know just actually drinks at home alone or, you know, actually is like an alcoholic ...
>
> INTERVIEWER: Yep. And what do you define as someone who's addicted?
>
> LING: It's kind of, they kind of look to that one thing as a solution for everything, yeah. So by drinking more than is healthy or drinking alone, and like when it gets in the way of other stuff.
>
> INTERVIEWER: Okay, what do you mean?
>
> LING: I don't know, like, if you had something on the next day and you just wanted to just drink so you just drank instead of going to whatever it was, or like, I don't know, like, if you had to drive but you drank anyway, stuff like that. Yeah, like, if it actually gets in the way of like your life instead of like being a fun addition.

Paul (22), too, thinks the meaning of drinking depends upon a range of factors such as age, occupation and conduct while intoxicated. Alcohol consumption, it seems, is not on its own a sign of any particular underlying state. When asked about what constitutes a drinking problem, he says:

> I don't know, well, [there's] a problem maybe [if] they lack self-control and then they're, you know, always passing out or being idiotically drunk every time we go out. But then that's hard because, you know, maybe you'd just say 'oh they're young, they're a uni student, they're getting it out of their system'. I guess you might start to think, yeah, it's more and more – well I don't know if it's a problem but it's not very dignified when it's a, an older person or something, like that when you think, well I hope that I might mature more.

For Paul, as for many other participants, the meaning of drinking is particularly heavily dependent upon the age of the drinker. It is certainly possible from this perspective to have a drinking problem, but identifying this problem as an attribute of the individual takes time; ageing must occur before the meaning of the conduct can be ascribed to the person rather than to the circumstances.

Placing these issues into a broader context, it is clear how indispensable social forces and processes are to discussions of the meaning and practice of drinking and the notion of an alcohol problem or an addiction. While our participants demonstrate some awareness of and willingness to invoke familiar markers of problematic drinking or addiction when asked, their comments often go much further than these statements, complicating them in important ways. The context or social environment of drinking is especially irreducible to such markers – it is the very stuff of what makes possible a judgement or diagnosis even as it also explains away conduct that might, if viewed through an expert lens, attract a diagnosis. Not only must context be taken into account when adjudging the meaning of drinking, it is often indivisible from the drinking itself. To return to the theoretical tools outlined earlier in relation to young women's drinking and Facebook, it seems drinking is, for young people, a complex assemblage, made of many constantly shifting, mutually constitutive phenomena, all of which must be considered if a judgement about the meaning of that drinking can be made. Gurnam (a 22-year-old man) and Ryan (23) offer good examples of these complex ways of understanding drinking. It is important to quote each at length in order to capture the nuances and complexities of their views.

As Gurnam's comments show, it is possible both to mobilise a relatively narrowly conceived idea of addiction to alcohol, and also to treat drinking, even heavy drinking, as a complex phenomenon with a range of meanings, causes and implications. During the course of his interview Gurnam frames binge drinking in quite subtle terms, trying over and again to communicate the social motivations and processes constituting it, at times resisting the interviewer's offers of rather more crude, if established, framings. In particular, Gurnam offers a very vivid account of the social processes behind the conviviality of binge drinking, first assenting to the proffered 'peer pressure' account, but also resisting it by rejecting the idea that the conduct is linked to the usual motivation ascribed to peer pressure: impressing friends. Gurnam also sees the sensation of intoxication as likely to be 'addictive', but his later comments on binge drinking suggest he is also aware that many people experience intoxication without falling prey to addiction.

> INTERVIEWER: Some people say that alcohol is addictive. What do you think about that?

GURNAM: I think it is addictive actually because people who consume it regularly do seem to have a sense [that] it's very normal to have it often. Like they can justify it by saying that, 'oh yeah you know, you're just having a few drinks, it's, it's harmless, you know', although it *is* harmful... So I would say that addiction is more [about] like justifying the consumption rather than... addiction itself. So like, you know, when you go to, when you go out you have a drink, but somehow the effect of the alcohol makes [you] want to have more and not stop, and the justification [is] that 'oh, you know, it's completely harmless, why can't I just keep having more and also more regularly?'

INTERVIEWER: Do you think it's denial, is that what it is?

GURNAM: Maybe denial. Denial of the fact that it is actually going to be harmful. I think some [... people] just enjoy the effect of alcohol. They don't want to accept that in the long run it will cause harm. So they are like, 'oh you know... I'm young, so I have every reason to enjoy it now, you know'...

INTERVIEWER: Right and what kind of harm are we talking about when we talk about the harm of alcohol?

GURNAM: I would say alcohol itself, I mean it is proven to cause liver damage over time, especially over a very regular consumption, so those kind of health issues can be avoided if you can, if you can control how much you're drinking. But... people who, who are kind of addicted to alcohol are able to justify this, or justify regular consumption saying that, 'oh yeah, you know, it's all right, I'm young now, you know.' It's not going to cause harm when in actual fact it does over a long time...

INTERVIEWER: Yeah and what, why do you think they would keep drinking?

GURNAM: Because... alcohol just gives the light-headed feeling that they, they – I would say that feeling is also maybe addictive probably – so they feel like, 'oh you know, after I had a stressful day or a stressful week why don't I drink alcohol to get the light-headed feeling?' So you know that, that kind of becomes like a routine, you know, 'I have a, I have a tough week, I match it up with a drink or a few drinks to lighten up the mood'. So if this [goes on] for a long time you just start to justify it as, you know, 'it's the only thing that's going to give me my, my stress relief', or something like that, and you kind of justify [it by saying] 'oh it's not causing harm, it's actually making it better. I kind of loosen up.'

INTERVIEWER: And how do you [tell] ... if someone's having drinking problem?

GURNAM: I think that a drinking problem just arises from how often they drink and the quantity they drink, you know like I, I would say that's the, the first point of measuring whether someone's having a drinking problem, you know. Did they buy drinks just from the store and just finish [them] off in like a few days or did they actually just have it ... once in a while?

[...]

INTERVIEWER: [What do you think is too often?] How many standard drinks maybe?

GURNAM: Maybe like two every day or three every day.

INTERVIEWER: Two every day or three every day?

GURNAM: And like on a regular basis, so.

INTERVIEWER: Regular basis: that might be a problem?

GURNAM: Yep, or even, maybe, like ten standard drinks on a weekend is also quite a lot I think on one night. So there have been instances where people do do that, so yeah.

In these comments Gurnam indicates a clear willingness to invoke alcohol addiction, citing the pharmacological effects of alcohol ('lightheadedness'), stress and reward as key drivers, but the circumstances under which this definition can be applied are less clear. Indeed, some way into his comments he shifts rather abruptly from a daily drinking model of the problem (and quite a low rate of consumption within it), to a binge drinking model of the problem. While it is not possible to establish retrospectively the reason for this sudden shift, we can speculate that one possible explanation is that the interviewer betrays surprise at the relatively modest volume of alcohol Gurnam nominates as problematic, and this leads him to seek firmer ground by emphasising larger volumes if lower frequency. The interviewer goes on to probe Gurnam's sense of the possible relationship between binge drinking and alcohol addiction.

INTERVIEWER: So, okay, the ten standard drinks in one sitting would be classified as binge drinking – so how does the idea of binge drinking fit with the idea of addiction for example?

GURNAM: I think binge drinking is more of like, 'oh, you know, I am doing it for the, you know ... popularity ... more than [because of an] alcohol problem', I would say.

INTERVIEWER: What's that, what do you mean?

GURNAM: Like, like binge drinking, you know everyone would be like, 'oh, you know, finish it, finish it, finish it' and, you know, they are just like, 'I am already a bit drunk so why not, I'll just gulp it down in one go' just to, you know, to fit in – not fit in but more like, 'I'm just into the mood' you know, 'I am in the mood right now' so that just happens. So I think that's more the mood rather than alcohol itself.

Here Gurnam seems to be attempting to distinguish the social meanings and forces around drinking from the pharmacological effects of alcohol alone. Similarly, he wants to distinguish the desire to join in with friends in creating and sustaining a fun mood from trying to impress them. As we see next, he goes on to accept the notion of peer pressure, if slightly hesitantly, but quickly rejects the idea that the drinking is just to do with 'fitting in'. Instead he is keen to offer a much more subtle account of motivations, adopting a particular narrative device, a first-person internal monologue style that allows him to represent intimate personal thoughts, to do so.

INTERVIEWER: Right, so mood or like getting into that kind of rowdy –

GURNAM: Yeah, not rowdy, more like . . . you are already, you already had a few drinks but people are like 'oh man', you know, you buy another drink but instead of having it slowly everyone's like 'finish it, finish it quickly' so you're just like ah, you know 'should I, should I not, ah, but everyone's enjoying [it so] let me just gulp it down in one go'. It's more the mood I would say.

INTERVIEWER: Is it more like, I guess, peer pressure and –

GURNAM: A bit, yeah, I would say, yeah.

INTERVIEWER: Yeah? And person trying to impress their friends or –

GURNAM: Not really impress, it's just more like, oh you know, 'I'm having fun as well' you know, 'I'm having fun, I'm not going to spoil the mood by not having it'.

Ryan's take on alcohol problems and addiction is rather different from Gurnam's, but it shares some important features in that he also often refuses to reduce drinking behaviour to narrow conceptions of the action of the substance or the vulnerable individual. For him, drugs, individuals and socialising are, at least in his own case, inextricable. Indeed, he dismisses very explicitly the idea of being addicted to drugs, proposing instead a considered and rather novel phenomenon – in our terms an assemblage of some abstraction and complexity – to which he is willing to say he is addicted. He is, he says, 'addicted to going out':

RYAN: Actually I studied what addiction meant years and years ago and, I think there was, there was the theory that it was like had five components or whatever, and . . . one of them was [that] you needed to have more each time or you needed to have more to sustain your addiction, but yeah, I mean, it's very hard I think to define what an addiction is. I mean, if you said to me 'don't drink for a year' I would struggle with that, but I don't think it would be because alcohol is addictive or, I mean, I don't think it would be because I was addicted to alcohol. I think it would be because I was, maybe addicted to going out, like I wanted to go out and I don't find going out a lot of fun when I'm not drinking or when I, yeah when I can't drink. I mean I know that it's addictive, I mean, I've been told that it's addictive but yeah, I mean, yeah . . .

INTERVIEWER: Right, I guess the whole using alcohol and pills and, and, is, is part of that going out?

RYAN: Yeah, definitely.

INTERVIEWER: So it's packaged in, so they go together and not separately?

RYAN: Yeah, definitely not.

In the follow-up question the interviewer tried to tease out whether the idea of addiction really applies to Ryan's feelings about going out, probing for more detail on what 'abstinence' from going out would mean, and the results are interesting:

INTERVIEWER: Right and [. . .] if . . . for whatever reason you could not go out, would you, what do you think would happen like to you mentally?

RYAN: Oh, I mean, if it was a decision that I made for my own choice I think I'd be fine with it . . . If it was forced upon me and I'd, you know, I don't think I'd cope with it very well. But I don't see, I mean, when I say 'going out' I don't just mean going out to a club or going out to a party. I mean going out with friends and even just going to a friend's house and drinking with them and that sort of thing. If I was not able to do that at all, yeah, I would not handle that very well.

INTERVIEWER: Right, so it's the companionship?

RYAN: Yeah, I mean, just seeing people, seeing friends and socialising and that whole thing.

Ryan's response performs several moves here. First he complicates his notion of addiction by making a clear distinction between choosing abstinence versus having it forced upon him. The experience of abstinence (and, we infer, of compulsion or desire) depends, he suggests, on the circumstances surrounding it. Then he seeks to clarify his terms, offering a broad definition of 'going out', apparently anticipating rather narrower notions confined to bars and clubs that might then lead back to narrower causal accounts of the role of alcohol and other drugs in social life and its problems. While he then seems to assent to the interviewer's summary that his addiction is about companionship, he – rather like Gurnam does in response to notions of 'peer pressure' and 'fitting in' – subtly turns the terms outwards again to broader, less bounded and more elusive concepts. Yes, companionship is part of it, but really it is about 'friends and socialising and that whole thing'. But Ryan is not quite satisfied with this articulation. He goes on to try again to explain his meaning, groping for a parallel to the conventional arrangement in which the source of the addiction, presumably illicit drugs, is outlawed. Here he seems to be moving towards a rather perceptive argument about the productivity of prohibition for sensations of addiction, but is sidetracked before concluding his point. As we will see, however, the turn in the conversation takes him back to a more conventional, that is, narrower, less diffuse, perspective on the meaning of drinking. For those not 'addicted to going out', drinking alone is clearly a sign of a problem, and genetics, it seems, might explain their compulsion.

RYAN: If I was, say I don't know, if I, if I had to relocate to a country where going out was illegal or something, and, you know, I had to spend all my time inside and, or something like that, I – and because I had to do it, yeah, I wouldn't be drinking, I wouldn't be taking drugs in the, just because I wouldn't be going out –

INTERVIEWER: Okay, so do you drink at home by yourself rather than, like, drinking wine with a meal –

RYAN: No, I never drink – I might have a drink before I go to meet friends, like if I'm getting ready or something I might have a beer – but I never drink by myself at home when I know I'm not going to go out [...]

INTERVIEWER: Right. What do you think about people who drink by themselves? Not just one can, one can or whatever but –

RYAN: Well [...] like one of my friends [...] would be drinking a bottle of wine a night and I don't think it's very healthy [...] or very good for her, yeah, and I think that's an addiction. And I've got another friend who yeah, who drinks by himself and, yeah, I don't think that's very good.

INTERVIEWER: Right and what, what makes, say this girl that you, you know what makes her addicted to alcohol?

RYAN: I'm not sure. I mean she, she really likes reading and taking a long bath and stuff, and I think a lot of the time she'll have a bath and read and drink wine in the bath, red wine and it'll be a way to I think prepare herself for getting, going to bed and stuff. I don't know why, like I don't know why – I've never felt the need to drink before going to bed so I think, yeah, I mean, she comes from a family of alcoholics I think, so maybe it's genetic and I think she's just been brought up around a lot of drinking.

Ryan's turn to genetics is interesting here. It seems that, in occurring at home, his friend's conduct lacks the social context in which broader understandings of the role of alcohol consumption can be framed and the sufficiency of simple notions of addiction to alcohol can be questioned. If all one is doing while drinking is reading and having a bath, the experience must be about the alcohol alone and the body's built-in vulnerability to it, even as all the elements he describes work together in his friend's apparent aim – preparation for sleep. This turn to genetics is all the more surprising given it emerges that Ryan too has a family history of 'alcoholism'.

INTERVIEWER: Right. And you know you mentioned about your grandfather, how has the fact that you know he had alcoholism made you think differently about alcohol?

RYAN: Well, no, because I was very young and I didn't, it didn't affect me. It affected my dad though and he, my dad doesn't drink beer now because my grandfather used to drink a lot of beer [...] he only drinks wine, and so I guess I haven't – I, I was never brought up around my grandfather so I never saw the, he, he was, yeah, quite a violent alcoholic I think, and so I was never exposed to that [...] I don't think it's had a big effect on me because yeah I never saw it so – and my dad he, he will drink probably a glass of wine a night but you would, you would not say, I would not say he was an alcoholic [...] that's the sort of drinking that I've been brought up with, to have a glass of wine, maybe two.

Here Ryan offers an account of drinking that differs again from the other two he has already outlined. In the first case, drinking is part of a larger assemblage – going out. In the second it constitutes a narrow problem, in his view probably the outcome of genetics. In this third case genetics do not appear to explain drinking in that, while his friend might have inherited alcoholism from the previous generation, Ryan's father did not do the same (that is, he did not inherit his own father's alcoholism). The origins of addiction and the elements that constitute it do not, it seems, follow any consistent pattern. What makes addiction, its origins and its character are, for Ryan, wholly contingent, subject to no consistent rules and not, we must conclude, amenable to the kinds of stabilisations so energetically pursued in the research analysed in the previous chapter. In particular, the narrow collateral reality of the 'environment' of alcoholism or addiction so consistently, if divergently, enacted in that discourse on alcohol addiction struggles for coherence here. This is perhaps unsurprising given the object described by Ryan in his use of the expression 'addiction' is so diffuse and multiple. The language of environment requires a certain kind of logic in which the alcohol problem, or let us say the 'elephant' so often invoked in the scientific debates, is a bounded and unified object outside of which exists a causal, or at minimum, contributing 'environment'. Where, instead, the addiction phenomenon is given so few clear edges – can in some cases be all about alcohol and genes, at others about social life in general and many diverse drivers – speaking of a readily identifiable *outside* or 'environment' makes little sense.

Perhaps the most vivid example of the kind of refusal to enact the narrow singular addiction phenomenon so ardently sought, if not achieved, in the research can be found in 23-year-old Naresh's account of the origins or causes of alcohol addiction. When asked how an addiction to alcohol occurs, he replies:

> You obviously have to control yourself, and think everything can be addictive, but you have to control, you have to see what's the right amount of alcohol, food et cetera [to consume] in a day. So it also depends on your background, your education, what kind of life you live and how, sometimes how successful you are in life, what kind of friends you have, what's your daily schedule, so all that sums up, and then, you know, you probably, some people get addicted [...] they drink every night. And also probably it also depends on the phase of your life [...] when you are in, you know, college and stuff, you're doing your graduate degree or some sort of thing, then you meet a lot of new people, you make friends every now and then and you don't have that pressure, you know, say you don't have a family [...] or you

> know you're on your own so you drink a lot. [...] Once you cross that phase, you start working fulltime, you, you know, think about getting married or starting a family, this sort of stuff, then you probably start drinking a bit less compared to your, that [earlier] phase. So I feel it also depends on that phase of life, and what kind of person you are, how, what's your background, how, what kind of friends you have. It also depends on [...] how much access to alcohol you have, so if you, if you've got friends, I mean, if you're living with three or four friends who, who are you know drinking a lot, then obviously you have got alcohol at your place, and when you've got alcohol at your place all the time you usually, you know [...] if I don't have beer at my home then I'll not specially go and buy [it] and then start drinking every day, but if, if I've got a slab at my place and, you know, I've got beer in my fridge every day, then I'll probably start drinking every day after I come home.

Here Naresh cites a strikingly comprehensive array of factors to be taken into consideration in how addiction develops: background, education, stage of life, friendships and social habits, availability. It is a sweeping account in which 'everything can be addictive' and every aspect of life can contribute to or act against addiction. Like Ryan, but perhaps even more explicitly, Naresh sketches such a diffuse and inclusive picture of the elements involved in the development of an addiction that notions of environment become unintelligible, as does any clear distinction between an alcohol problem and an addiction. In these respects Naresh's account reflects, but also exceeds, others given in the interviews. Like almost all participants he is able to articulate a view on the features of drinking that might constitute a problem or even an addiction. Indeed, as already noted, criteria for judging drinking were offered almost universally. If one were to assume that expert discourse unproblematically trickles down to public discourse, these articulations could be interpreted merely as echoes of the research debates that have raged across the last five decades (analysed in the previous chapter). Importantly, however, many of the participants simultaneously demonstrate a disinclination to simplify reality in the way the researchers whose work we analysed aim to do. They do not, for example, enact such criteria as independently decisive or reliable. Yes, Ryan's friend might be caught in the grip of her genetic fate, but his father was not. Yes, if Naresh is not yet burdened with family and work responsibilities, he might fall into the habit of drinking heavily, but only if there is a slab of beer in the house already – he would not make a special trip to buy it. Addiction is made, we are told, if not always expressly, out of the manifold intra-actions (Barad 2003) of a dizzying array of phenomena. When circumstances, friendships and social patterns change, it follows, so do the drinking habits, even when they have come to possess what might seem a life of their own. One might be tempted to demur here, to argue that addiction is precisely that which defies change, that persists even where everything else is undergoing change or, to adopt the conventional cautionary register, collapsing around one. Yet this would be to deny the very clear sense in which addictions do indeed change, to deny that, for reasons little researched and poorly understood perhaps because this change is precluded precisely by the core notion of addiction as *stasis*, the very repetition with which addiction is identified has always already within it the seeds of change (Fraser & valentine 2008).

Conclusion: Assembling drinking

In summing up the material analysed in this chapter and the arguments we have made, it is first important to emphasise that our intention is not to idealise the perspectives on alcohol consumption and addiction offered by our participants. As is probably clear by now, these perspectives throw up as many questions as they answer, take as many detours via familiar metaphors as they do paths to new ways of seeing. But it is certainly the case that the ways of seeing they articulate diverge quite markedly from (even as they reflect the same struggles in) the research debates about alcohol. In particular they suggest that the collateral realities so energetically if inconclusively constituted in the science – the stable anterior object of problem drinking, the 'environment' as 'influence on' this anterior object, the erasure of caveats and qualifications in the production of the realities of dependence and pathology – do not wash or hold together especially well for the young people the science seeks to comprehend and represent. And it must be said that, given most of the research and popular criteria for judgements about drinking are social in substance (how relationships are affected, how work is managed, the appropriateness of the drinking to the occasion, whether responsibilities are being met), this reticence to stabilise or render narrowly the notion of alcohol addiction seems to us only sensible. Just as social expectations about appropriate occasions, personal responsibilities, professional conduct and social relationships change over time, so too must individual status as a 'normal' or 'healthy' drinker or a problem drinker or alcoholic. As we know well from the many important historical studies long on the record in this field, the defining features of alcoholism and other such problems vary considerably over time, indeed in a past only barely beyond living memory, they did not exist in any meaningful sense at all (Levine 1978; Room 2003).

To return to the theoretical resources this book draws upon, we should not be unduly surprised by the variations in accounts of drinking – in the realities of drinking and the collateral realities enacted to stabilise these realities – visible in the research and those of the youth population with which they are increasingly concerned. As John Law (2011, 165) suggests, the kinds of variation we described in the last two chapters, both within research discourse and between experts and the objects of their knowledges, can be seen as effects of differing needs or requirements for 'institutional survival'. Just as medical and public health realities are made and remade amid the shifting connections and forces of the institutional assemblages in which they find themselves at different times (the negotiations between parties necessary to producing a new *DSM*, the imperative of progress built into the ethos of science and thus the neuroscience of addiction, and so on), so too are young people's accounts shaped as the meanings being made around, and the lived experiences of, youth also change in relation to institutional requirements (as suggested in the forces identified in Measham 2007). In closing, then, instead of trying to resolve or render consistent these variations, our inclination is to reiterate the value of seeing realities as 'performed', and of the notion of the assemblage. In particular, in that our interview participants make a vivid case for the irreducibility of drinking and its problems, we consider the assemblage an especially productive alternative to the existing (apparently unexamined) ontology mobilised in the influential research we explored – a realist one in which a bounded object, an elephant we are sometimes told, has wandered into our community and must be identified, defined and examined in all its parts to produce a comprehensive picture of the whole animal so that we can most effectively respond to it. Put this way, the elephant metaphor is in fact wonderfully productive. Not only does it raise questions about the origins of this animal, it also leads us to wonder about its place in the community, its attributes and its value. We do not, these days at least, tend to think stray elephants should be destroyed, even when they trample crops and terrorise residents. In any case, as our discussion suggests, there is no elephant; alternatively, if there is an elephant there is also a whale, a giant redwood, a meteor and any number of other massively manifesting phenomena of addiction. But more than this, the object, however big or sprawling, is not singular. If it can be said to coalesce into a coherent beast at all, this is only for a moment, and this beast is never as neat or unified as the figurative creatures to which we might wish to compare it. Instead it is unstable and messy, enacted in many and diverse constituents beyond the familiar parts we might expect of the creature we think we recognise, just as is Brown and Gregg's Facebooking binge drinking. This matters because, so long as we wish to pursue the familiar habit of constituting labile objects such as addiction as singular and stable, we will be obliged to exclude from their ontology much that, at any given moment is – temporarily rather than permanently – actually *a part of it*. We will treat these elements as external to the object in our attempt to reify the object, and in so doing we will necessarily oversimplify it, with serious consequences. This, in the end, is the merit of the assemblage – it allows more to be held at once in the constitution of objects or problems. As we will see in the section that follows this one, this simplification is underway in the most energetic of modes in relation to a beast possibly even more sprawling and indeed indispensable than the elephant of drinking: food and eating.

6
Junk: The Neuroscience of Food Addiction and Obesity

Can food be understood as a kind of drug? This depends on the way in which the notion of the 'drug' is itself defined. Drugs can be seen in terms of Mary Douglas's definition of pollution – as matter out of place (Keane 2002). In this sense, the category of drugs is an entirely political one: it contains all substances the consumption of which attracts social opprobrium at a given time. Indeed, foods such as sugar, fat and even staples such as bread are coming to be described as drugs in some contexts. Due in large part to the current climate of fear about obesity (Campos et al. 2005; Monaghan 2005; Stephenson & Banet-Weiser 2007), but also reflecting a much longer concern about obesity and addictive eating (Parr & Rasmussen 2012), some foods are no longer just foods; they are increasingly framed as illicit substances, especially for people classified as overweight. As Eve Sedgwick (1993) has noted, anorexia, bulimia and obesity are all now open to definition as dysfunctions of control, as addictive behaviour. How are these new concerns about junk food, health and compulsion remaking realities of drug use and addiction? Categories of overweight and obesity capture so many individuals, pathologise so large a portion of the population, that their association with compulsivity and addiction must surely demand some drift from margin to centre for those concepts. In this third section of the book, our aim is to continue our trajectory of enquiry across fields of addiction attribution, leaving behind the highly stigmatised domain of methamphetamine use and the traditionally normalised, but now increasingly suspect, domain of alcohol consumption to explore food, a basic requirement of life that is increasingly portrayed as just as risky as the most potent of illicit drugs. In doing so we explore food and obesity as a case study of changing ideas about addiction, asking how this new area of public concern is reframing addiction.

Drawing on an analysis of scientific journal articles that link obesity and addiction, in this first chapter in the section we examine the assumptions that drive such linkages and their implications and effects.[1] As the articles make clear, where obesity is linked to addiction it is increasingly accounted for via neuroscientific theories of behaviour, and little attention is paid to the *DSM* and its criteria for addiction or dependence. The brain's reward system is cited, along with the operations of endogenous opioids and cannabinoids, to enact 'excessive' eating as addictive behaviour, and 'highly palatable' or junk foods as akin to conventional drugs – that is, intrinsically addictive in their chemistry. In the process, a range of phenomena are made. In John Law's terms (2011), numerous important collateral realities are produced. 'Drug addiction' is referred to as though no controversy exists over its interpretation, and criteria for diagnosis as though they are entirely stable, no longer subject to revision. As Chapter 1 makes clear, this is far from the case. Likewise, 'drugs' are often produced as a homogenous group, the attributes of which, contrary to dominant accounts of drug addiction, are seen to warrant no differentiation. Other collateral realities produced include that of the body itself: where obesity is explained by the actions of the brain, and susceptible types are posited, individual tendencies to cycle between fatter and thinner over time are largely erased and the body is treated as unchanging and stable. Similarly, in a move reminiscent of the reduction of the social contexts of drinking to environment-as-family, complex social and cultural aspects of food and eating are reduced and scientised as 'environment'.

Through these processes of stabilisation and simplification, the limitations of such accounts of food, the body, health and well-being are exposed. Indeed, in our view food and eating demonstrate even more clearly than does methamphetamine or alcohol consumption the limits of neuroscientific accounts of complex, socially embedded practices. We must ask why addiction appeals so strongly as an explanatory framework here, when the epidemiology of overweight and obesity would suggest the processes at work are as normal as any that produce normatively slim bodies. Does the neuroscience of obesity require the normalisation of addiction? If so, what are the implications of this?

The social science of overeating and obesity

This discussion of the development of scientific and public health accounts of obesity sets off from the critical social science literature on obesity rather than from the literature on addiction or drugs, mainly because it offers important insights into a set of fears that have only recently become cast in the language of addiction.[2] Over the last decade intense concern has developed in the West about what has been characterised as an obesity epidemic. This concern has been accompanied by equally intense debates over the validity of this characterisation, with some critics arguing that while body size is increasing, rates do not constitute an epidemic and, in any case, research is yet to conclusively demonstrate that obesity is universally harmful. Social scientists have raised a range of questions and concerns about the terms of the obesity debate and its broader validity (for example, see Campos et al. 2005; Monaghan 2005; Lobstein 2006; Stephenson & Banet-Weiser 2007). Scholars have contested the epidemiology behind claims of an obesity epidemic, questioned the negative health judgements being made about fat and attempted to locate discussion of the meaning of weight, fat, health and fitness in a social context and in a more cautious approach to medicalisation than is found in the public health and medical literature. An early critical approach to the proliferating discourse on obesity can be found in Gard and Wright's (2001) article, 'Managing uncertainty: Obesity discourses and physical education in a risk society'. The article focuses on the implications of the debate for physical education for children and argues that a kind of premature certainty has been generated about the effects and implications of obesity. Ulrich Beck's notion of the risk society is used to explore the rise of obesity discourse and to argue that obesity is now seen as a risk of modern Western life. Gard and Wright point out that the language of risk introduces the idea that danger can be quantified, and they challenge this idea particularly in relation to the body, arguing that contrary to recent efforts:

> It may well be that the body is not an object that lends itself at all well to rational quantification . . . we need to see scientific uncertainty about the body not as a curse but as confirmation that we are not machines. (2001, 546–547)

An equally critical approach to the obesity epidemic is found in an article by Monaghan (2005). Part of a group of three articles on obesity published in the same issue of *Social Theory & Health*, it questions the science behind the 'war on fat', casting doubt on the perceived epidemic of excess weight among UK men. As Monaghan puts it:

> The highly publicised 'obesity debate' often focuses upon proposed 'solutions' to a taken-for-granted 'problem' (or apocalyptic problem

> in the making) rather than questioning the construction of fatness as a massive public health problem that should be tackled. (2005, 303)

The point being made here is twofold: rates of overweight are not necessarily as high as is claimed, and the effects of overweight on health are also uncertain. Monaghan does not argue that high weight is never harmful to health (although he does query the assumption that it is *always* harmful to health). Instead, he calls for debate that refuses the polarisation of health along slim/fat lines and observes that '[s]pace exists here for productive dialogue without being forced to adopt an essentialist either/or position that is intertwined with other questionable dichotomies' (2005, 303).

This insightful non-dualist approach characterises the article as a whole. As with Gard and Wright's approach to the non-rational, it is careful to avoid either denigrating the usual targets (emotion, fat, the body) or inappropriately valorising them (as some have argued is not helpful – see below for more). Instead, Monaghan's choice of language often consciously disrupts our usual assumptions about the alignments between bodies, body size and value. For instance, he locates the obesity debate in a growing horror of fat based not on incontrovertible evidence but on social norms, writing 'I question the very public degradation of fatness and, in suggesting possible ways forward, accord due weight to the social body concerning matters of health and illness' (2005, 305).

This form of words seeks to reframe 'weight' by reminding us of the sense in which it can confer authority and value as much as stigma in Western discourse. Towards the end of the article, Monaghan again draws on metaphors of food, fat and the body to subtly illustrate the related point that these phenomena also operate as potent objects of anxiety and uncertainty:

> ...because the war against obesity cannot be divorced from economics (there are obviously big fat profits to be made), it is legitimate to ask interested parties on which side is their bread buttered and whether they can afford to leave it without fear of going hungry? (2005, 312)

In this extract, the expression 'big fat profits' reminds us of the association between fat and excess and greed in Western discourse, while the reference to bread and butter also reminds us that food (even those foods now of ambiguous health status) still operates as positive metaphors for the essentials of life. Similarly, the reference to 'going hungry' points to the centrality of food and the body (in the sensation of hunger) to notions of well-being, risk and deprivation. All these uses serve to highlight the intensity with which we invest food and body size with social and emotional meaning. As such, they suggest that simplistic understandings of and solutions to overeating, such as those that focus on rational calculations of food input and energy expenditure, are unlikely to ever find lasting purchase in decisions about food and activity in daily life.

In keeping with this nuanced approach to the symbolics of bodies and fat, Monaghan also pays attention to the operations of power and stigma in the debate, noting that 'obesity epidemic talk' is inseparable from social, cultural, political and economic concerns and therefore the exercise of power (2005, 309). Likewise, he recognises that body fat invokes and relies on a series of potent social and cultural concepts and attributes, and that these are the source of our negative views on it. In particular, he argues that body fat is 'a deeply personalised corporeal marker for inferior social status' (2005, 310), thereby challenging the assumption that body fat prompts our disgust simply because it is unhealthy and a sign of personal weakness. Indeed, the emphasis on fat and its denigration as deeply personal in itself extends the 'problem' of body size well beyond those formulations that rely on simplistic rational correctives.

Like Monaghan, Paul Campos and colleagues (2005) also argue that concern about obesity is unnecessarily high in that it is not supported by evidence. In brief, the article challenges several dominant assumptions: (1) overweight and obesity have reached epidemic proportions; (2) overweight and obesity lead to increased mortality rates; (3) overweight and obesity lead to increased morbidity rates and (4) significant long-term weight loss is a realistic attainable goal that will improve health. Compelling alternative interpretations of the data are presented, all of which frame the debate's interlocutors as inappropriately obsessed with fat and its putative harmful effects. Again like Monaghan, Campos et al. refer often to 'the war on fat' (for example, 57, 58) and offer a range of reasons for the widespread misinterpretation of data and the accompanying 'rhetoric', arguing that it is driven by 'cultural and political factors' (55). In short, they propose a primarily economic explanation for the production of anti-fat discourse, but combine this with references to the role of 'ideology', 'anxieties' and 'morality'.

Campos et al. (2005, 58) also draw out the important relationship between negative judgements about obesity and negative attitudes towards minorities and the poor, and situate these in broader social and political issues such as immigration and the economy. The authors summarise the causes of what they describe as a moral panic about obesity as '...propagating the idea of an "obesity epidemic" [that] furthers the political and economic interests of certain groups, while doing immense damage to those whom it blames and stigmatises' (2005, 59).

While there is certainly some accuracy in this account, its emphasis on intention (to propagate, to profit, to stigmatise) misses an opportunity to take account of the complexity in perceptions of fat, the body and virtue in the West and the meanings and emotions surrounding them (see Thomas et al. [2008] for empirical research on fat stigma and emotions, and Fraser et al. [2010] on the limits of the notion of 'moral panic' for obesity). These multiple, tangled factors make a critical contribution to understandings of obesity and to the proliferation of anti-obesity discourse, and need to be attended to if we are to consider most effectively new trends in treating obesity as the product of food addiction.

Emma Rich and John Evans (2005) take an important step in their discussion of this debate, according emotions substantial power in shaping the way obesity is thought. Unlike other researchers they explicitly acknowledge the need to consider emotions, those of affected individuals and those operating in the broader social context, more thoroughly. Bethan Evans (2006) also alludes to complex emotional forces at work in how obesity is understood, referring for instance to the role of guilt in reactions to it. She notes that the emotional aspects of eating and body size are largely ignored in policy, save to list shame and guilt as causes of overeating. She advocates a different approach to body size that puts subjectivity and emotion at the centre of designations of well-being by focusing on 'an alternative, non-medical reading of obese or fat bodies where being healthy is about *feeling* healthy...' (2006, 265).

These contributions go some way towards locating obesity and fat as social and cultural concepts, establish ng that knowledge about the fat body, even apparently objective epidemiological knowledge, is itself shaped by long-standing culturally specific fears and assumptions about food and fat bodies. In this literature we also begin to see the traces of many points of crossover between fears about overeating and fears about drug addiction: ideas about personal weakness and lack of control, stigma and its disproportionate distribution among minorities and the poor, even some obvious echoes in the expression 'the war on fat'. However, such links and the complexities to which they relate are not exhausted by this set of issues. For more detailed, sophisticated analyses of the meaning of the fat body, it is useful to turn to the feminist literature.

Feminism and the fat body

As the preceding section suggests, obesity and the many political, public health and medical responses to it need to be understood as enacted within complex nets of meaning, subjective experience and social relations, all informed by normative concepts of gender, race and class. This is also true of the powerfully abjected central object of the debate, fat itself. Here, feminists have made a distinctive contribution to understanding the meaning of obesity and the responses and effects that attend it. Two decades ago, influential critic Susan Bordo (1993) made a now classic argument about the meaning of fat and the way in which it operates as a gendered figure for ambiguity, permeability and unruliness. Utilising Mary Douglas's insight that 'the "microcosm" – the physical body – may symbolically reproduce central vulnerabilities and anxieties of the "macrocosm" – the social body' (1993, 186), Bordo argued that the contemporary attachment to the slender, toned body relates to concerns about the '"correct" management of desire' (1993, 187) and the containment of threatening and unruly flesh. In her account, the bulging body is 'a metaphor for anxiety about internal processes out of control' (1993, 189). Much more recently, Samantha Murray (2005, 266) has argued that we are 'asked... to read the fat body as a site of moral and physical decay'. LeBesco and Braziel (2001, 3) also draw attention to the meanings of fat, noting that the fat body invokes 'reckless excess, prodigality, indulgence, lack of restraint, violation of order and space, transgression of boundary'. While women have long been a particular target of these fears in part because the attributes described also speak to fears about the feminine (Bordo 1993, 206), Western social and cultural frameworks now encourage all of us to contain and control the body. While the 'fat woman' has registered as particularly problematic, fat also implicitly works to undermine or discredit masculinity. Fat, wherever it materialises, feminises and casts into doubt the rationality of anyone affected, including 'fat' men and 'fat' children.

Feminist challenges to normative and proscriptive representations of body size have also included celebrations of the non-normative 'fat' body. In their edited volume, *Bodies out of Bounds* (2001), Braziel and LeBesco aim to 'reconceptualise and reconfigure corpulence' (LeBesco & Braziel 2001, 1), challenging phobic and simplistic responses to fat bodies. According to Murray (2005), 'the fat pride' movement invites women to view their otherwise denigrated bodies with pride. As Saguy and Riley put it (2005, 870), 'fat activism... reclaim[s] the word fat'. Some critics have, however, queried the move to frame fat as resistance.

Yancey et al. (2006) challenge the feminist focus on the perils of the slender body, arguing that fat is negatively affecting the health of the least advantaged women and that feminists are failing to address the social inequalities manifest in weight. Probyn (2008, 402) has questioned the 'semiotic reversal' suggested in the reclamation of fat. For Probyn, 'there is something seriously wrong with an analysis that leaves untouched the socioeconomic structures that are producing ever larger bodies' (2008, 402). For these scholars, feminist celebrations or revaluations of weight against the medical and social control of bodies fail to take account of the economic and gendered inequities of fat and obesity. Critical examinations of the 'global obesity' phenomenon suggest that body shapes and sizes reflect global patterns of resource distribution as well as individual social locations. Bodies materially reveal what Probyn describes as 'the immense changes in global flows of capital and agribusiness, which are putting millions out of traditional work and forcing them into cities' (2008, 402). While Probyn's critique raises important issues to do with disadvantage and access to health, it has been criticised for taking the 'obesity epidemic' for granted (Kirkland 2011).

Bordo (1993) identified the complex gendered negotiations of social power in fat and slender bodies, in loose and taut flesh. Her suggestion that there were 'two different symbolic functions of body shape and size – the designation of social position, such as class status or gender role; and the outer indication of the spiritual, moral or emotional state of the individual' (1993, 187) – drew attention to the need to recognise the complexity of the meanings attributed to fat, the body, food and eating. Murray's account (2005) of her brief immersion in the fat pride movement and of the strong negative response others have to her body weight offers a good example of this kind of recognition. As she contends, 'every time the fat woman hides her eating from others ... she is really eating other people's disgust at her body' (2005, 217). As with Bordo's observations about the symbolic function of fat, Murray's work points to the profound, intricate and powerful social and cultural forces expressed in food and flesh beyond the 'health' or otherwise of individual overweight bodies. And, like the broader social science literature discussed earlier, the observations she and other feminists make are striking for the links they suggest between the fat body and the addicted body, and between judgements about the morality of consumption and dependence.

It is on these broad social science and explicitly feminist literatures that the analysis conducted here is built. What is obesity and on what foundations are our fears about it based? What is fat? How does it function symbolically? What about food? Is it just fuel, is it a drug, or does its meaning run deeper and resonate more widely than this? These literatures offer (at least) four critical observations that form the basis for this analysis:

1. the 'obesity epidemic' should not be taken for granted;
2. fears about overweight and obesity are informed by a range of factors – commercial forces, historical concepts of the proper body, and gender and class norms – beyond the 'pure science' of physiology, endocrinology and other health sciences;
3. fat should be understood as profoundly social and symbolic, as should food; and
4. the politics of eating, fat and obesity are complex and cannot be easily reduced either to simple health concerns or to ideas of resistance and self-determination.

Clearly, obesity, fat and food cannot be lifted from their social and political circumstances if we are to understand their significance and account for their effects convincingly. Indeed, any analysis of the scientific literature on obesity needs such insights to allow critical purchase on issues otherwise presented as incontrovertible facts of value-free scientific method.

Taking on these lessons from the critical social science literature on obesity and fat requires an approach able to treat the object of analysis as social, as performed or enacted by complex social and political forces, as well as fully material. As in previous chapters, John Law's work on collateral realities is again useful here. All phenomena (such as the body or the disease of obesity) are, according to this approach, *made in practice* rather than given in nature. How does this enactment of realities, this making in practice, work? As we will see, different strategies enact different realities at different moments according to different needs. This, Law (2011, 165) observes, is a requirement of 'institutional survival'.

There is much to take from Law's approach in analysing the medical journal articles collected for this chapter. The analysis is based on a corpus of 40 articles collected from key peer-reviewed obesity and addiction journals (*Addiction, Obesity Reviews* and *International Journal of Obesity*), as well as articles chosen from a range of other scientific journals for their dual focus on addiction and obesity. The resulting collection provides a broad overview of the developing addiction approach to obesity, and within this the turn to the neuroscience of addiction. As we will see, increasingly conceived as the effect of a form of addiction (food addiction), obesity is linked in the scientific literature more and more directly with the dominant neuroscience account of addiction as brain disease, and individual conduct as the direct effect of brain chemistry. Particular collateral realities are enacted in these accounts – realities of addiction, drugs, the body and the social. The discussion that follows considers the relations at work to constitute particular realities of obesity, how the stability of these realities is achieved and maintained, and the processes or strategies by which this stabilising work is simultaneously obscured or 'washed away' (Law 2011, 171). Are there gaps and tensions within the neuroscientific account and between it and lay accounts of overweight and obesity? If so, how do these affect the realities enacted? In all these questions the role of collateral realities is, following Law, crucial. In his view, 'it is the endless enactment of collateral realities that tends to hold things steady' (2011, 172). We would add that, where criticism is warranted, one or more of the collateral realities holding a particular reality stable may offer a valuable entry point – that is, may prove vulnerable to destabilisation. In turn, other linked realities may be destabilised. As Law reminds us:

> [W]hatever is not contested and, more particularly, whatever lies *beyond the limits of contestability* is that which operates most powerfully to do the real. And it is this, to be sure, that is the technique that lies at the heart of common sense realism. It is the enactment of collateral realities that turns what is being done in practice into what necessarily *has* to be [emphasis in the original]. (2011, 174)

Our aim in this chapter is to examine four key collateral realities produced in the scientific enactment of obesity (addiction, drugs, the 'environment' and the body), to think through how these realities work to constitute and hold stable a new object of addiction. In the chapter that follows this one, we build on this analysis to assess how these realities fare in the leap from the institutional context of scientific knowledge practices to public enactments of overeating and obesity.

Repeating addiction?

Probably the most significant reality enacted collaterally to the central phenomenon of obesity in the scientific literature collected here is that of 'addiction' itself. Literature linking obesity with addiction began to emerge in the early 1980s and has grown unevenly over time, appearing in small clusters often with many years' gap in between. Quite different accounts of obesity occur across this temporal spread, drawing on changing accounts of addiction itself. This is one of the challenges or opportunities of linking obesity and addiction – neither phenomenon enjoys conceptual stability. Just as obesity has been defined and measured differently across the last 30 years or so since it began emerging as a significant public health issue, so too, of course, has addiction itself. As earlier chapters have made clear, definitions of addiction have been contested vigorously over time. The *DSM* has reviewed its criteria and terminology several times. Movements in mental health have influenced the emphasis definitions have taken, shifting between psychoanalytic notions to social psychological notions of trauma and social determinants, to, more recently, the neuroscientific accounts of the vulnerable brain explored here. The aetiology, attributes and implications of addiction have long been and remain heavily contested, and a range of different treatment modalities and responses (abstinence, harm reduction and so on), often accompanied by intense dispute, have developed. Yet this variation across time (along with persistent multiplicity at any given time) tends to be downplayed, at times 'washed away', in the scientific literature on obesity as addiction.

In some publications, usually earlier ones dating before the advent of the neuroscience of addiction, definitions of addiction are subjected to close scrutiny, and arguments for expanding them to include eating are made. In such cases the commitment to a single comprehensive definition is clear. In other cases, the stability and utility of existing definitions are taken for granted. Is obesity the effect of addiction? This commonly asked question acts to produce addiction as a single, stable and self-evident object whether or not the authors conclude in the affirmative or the negative. Marks (1990), for example, offers a very confident (in some respects narrow, in others extremely broad) definition of addiction in his formulation of the similarities between drug addiction and what he calls behavioural addictions such as 'overeating (bulimia)': 'Addiction denotes repetitive routines that aim to obtain chemicals and, less often, routines without that aim. The latter are behavioural addictions' (1990, 1389). Here addiction is defined narrowly in that it must be about repetition, but broadly in that it embraces anything characterised by routine. As is suggested by the publication date (1990), this article does not draw in any detail on neuroscientific accounts of addiction. It does make reference to questions about the role of dopamine in the brain, but, it says, such questions offer scientists only 'tantalising clues' at this stage. Instead, the article takes the WHO definition of 'dependence syndrome' as its starting point to argue for a more global definition that embraces compulsive acts or thoughts beyond those directly related to drugs. Here we can see the beginnings of contemporary interest in linking addiction to food, and the use of a particular marker of addiction (repetition) to open the way for this linkage. Marks' (1990, 1389) opening observation (which cites breathing, eating, drinking and other bodily functions) that '[l]ife is a series of addictions and without them we die', places repetition squarely at the centre of *both* addiction and healthy living. In the process, it enacts a collateral reality of drug addiction as repetitive drug consumption, and suggests that, debates about behaviour aside, a stable agreed-upon category of drug addiction exists.

At the same time that drug addiction is enacted as a single stable object here – as repetitive consumption of a drug – its meaning is also given a novel emphasis in that traditional ideas of repetitive consumption and dependence as purely aberrant are disrupted, framed instead as normal, indeed in many cases essential. Food is, of course, something we must all consume regularly and consistently. In this sense, repetition is the basis of life itself and as such we are all 'dependent' – upon breathing, eating and so on. Consequently, Marks suggests that notions of food addiction cannot rely on repetitive consumption for diagnosis. Even repetitive consumption of 'bad' ('highly palatable' junk) foods – discussed in the next section – cannot provide the basis for diagnosis in that body weight must exceed levels classified as healthy before concern about food intake is warranted. In other words, some people's ability to eat chocolate and chips each day without exceeding weight injunctions rules out repetition or habit as in itself a basis on which to define food addiction. Instead, the notion of 'bingeing' is given more emphasis (in Marks' article, this is bulimia), an idea we have seen emerge in recent times as acute or episodic consumption in relation to other drugs such as methamphetamine and alcohol (see Chapters 2 and 4).

Writing approximately ten years after Marks, Orford (2001) also argues for a global definition of addiction, and for the inclusion of non-drug-related phenomena (he cites gambling, eating and sex), again enacting a particular reality of addiction in the process. Citing a 17th-century sermon, he argues that despite many debates, a simple definition of addiction is possible and desirable, and it is one that serves a broader notion of 'appetite' equally well. According to this sermon (cited in 2001, 16), addiction can be identified when

> by long usage, an activity that was originally pleasurable has become a 'necessity'... a strong craving is part of the experience; and... despite the many harms that it has brought, neither the

exercise of reason nor encouragement from others have been sufficient to bring about control.

Here, as in Marks' definition, repetition occupies an important place, leading to a shift from choice to necessity, and along with it an absence or loss of control. Craving, a concept familiar to diet and weight loss discourse, is also foregrounded here, as it is in much of this literature. In this way, longer-standing enactments of addiction aimed at emblematic substances such as alcohol and heroin, and emphasising the problem of repetition as daily use, are remade to emphasise aspects of diagnosis more suited to the particular features of eating and overeating.

Other research, notably more recently published work, departs from the explicit call to redefine addiction made in these articles. Instead, it treats definitions of addiction drawn from the drug field as self-evident, erasing (or washing away) instability and uncertainty as it does so. Davis, for example, aims to identify psychological and biological risk factors for overeating, rehearsing the debate about the links between eating and addiction, and noting that overeating and 'addiction disorders such as drug abuse... both activate the same reward systems' (2009, S49). According to Davis, they have 'comparable clinical features, such as their escalating compulsion, the symptoms of tolerance and withdrawal, and the overwhelming cravings that contribute to repeated relapses after periods of restraint or abstinence' (2009, S49).

Here the clinical features of drug addiction are treated as consistent, self-evident and beyond controversy. As we have already demonstrated, assumptions of this kind do not have a strong basis; indeed, debate about the presence or otherwise of elements such as tolerance and withdrawal remains vigorous and in some important cases, such as that of methamphetamine, it is rare to find withdrawal included at all.

In another article (Gearhardt et al. 2011), the enactment of food addiction's collateral reality – drug addiction – goes a step further. Discussing the addictiveness of food, the authors state that '[f]ood shares multiple features with addictive drugs' especially in their effect on neurocircuitry. The article goes on to propose that '[f]oods and abused drugs may induce similar sequelae, including craving, continued use despite negative consequences and diminished control over consumption' (2011, 1208) and suggests that given this, 'lessons learned from drug addiction' (2011, 1208) can be applied to obesity policy, prevention and treatment. Claiming that neuroscientific accounts of addiction have achieved progress beyond accounts that hold individual drug users responsible for their actions, the article invokes the common trope of the hijacked brain, asserting that this trope may also aid understanding of overweight and obesity. Here, as in Davis's article, the nature of drug addiction (craving, continued use, diminished control) is taken for granted. Its features are then attributed to 'food problems' and obesity with such a degree of conviction that transfer of policy and practice from the drug field is considered desirable. While the article adopts a provisional tone at points ('[f]oods and abused drugs *may* induce similar sequelae [emphasis added]'), the overall aim of the article belies this caution. It proceeds as though drug addiction is well understood and its features agreed by consensus, and it enacts drug policy, prevention and treatment as so successful as to warrant emulation.

Elsewhere, similar assumptions about the utility of drug addiction responses prompt explicit calls for the classification of overeating and obesity as addiction disorders so that they can then be treated using the principles and practices of conventional addiction treatment. Davis and Carter (2009, 5), for example, argue that although abstinence-based treatments are not viable for eating disorders, and CBT is not effective for a substantial proportion of patients, the 'implicit message' sent by a diagnosis of addiction – that affected individuals 'may be fighting a strong neurobiological drive to overeat in an environment that exploits these urges' – could help foster a 'therapeutic sense of self-empathy' and encourage participation in addiction treatment. Interestingly, this portrayal of food addiction does not approximate the way drug addiction is generally understood as closely as might be expected given the article's conviction that the two would usefully be classified together. While some responses to drug addiction do exhibit a degree of tolerance and sympathy for addicts, there is little evidence that individuals diagnosed with drug addiction emerge with an equally exculpatory view of themselves as 'fighting a strong neurological urge' 'exploited' by their 'environment'.

Davis and Carter (2009, 6) also promote treatment by arguing that '[t]here is also now a range of available medications for each of the major classes of drugs which, in combination with psychotherapy or counselling, have been effective in reducing the likelihood of relapse'. This remark is as unexpected as their previous statement, both because it is difficult, at least at this point in time, to imagine overeaters willingly being prescribed most of the actually rather limited (and unspecified) range of relevant medications presumably included here (opioid replacement pharmacotherapies such as methadone or buprenorphine? naltrexone?) and also because the language tends to overstate their effectiveness and acceptability, even among existing target groups. As do Gearhardt's comments, this turn to the benefits of drug addiction models for the sake of treatment enacts addiction treatments as broadly effective and successful. On the contrary, just as the attributes of addiction, and the criteria by which it can be meaningfully diagnosed, remain contested, so do assessments of the effectiveness of current treatments (Ritter & Lintzeris 2004).

To sum up, discussions of the relationship between overeating and drug addiction remake addiction in particular ways (craving, bingeing) that allow the inclusion of overeating and other 'behavioural' phenomena in the category of addiction. Collateral to this remaking are at least two further (highly politically charged) realities: first, the enactment of drug addiction as the object of consensus, its attributes as beyond doubt, and second, a notably optimistic view of drug addiction policy measures and treatment responses as uncontroversially successful and therefore meriting extension to food.

Doing 'drugs'

Just as the scientific literature tends to stabilise the concept of addiction, it also stabilises another key concept, that of 'drugs'. As Derrida (1993, 2) has observed, popular mobilisations of the idea of 'drugs' tend to conflate all substances, treating it as a 'buzzword'. While this tendency can also be found at times in public health and treatment responses to drug use, different drugs, especially legal and illegal, are also carefully distinguished, and different effects on the mind and the body are ascribed to each. Within the neuroscientific account of drug addiction, which draws on the brain's 'reward system' to explain addiction, different drugs are also seen as having different effects. Some, such as cannabis or heroin, are said to directly mimic or replace endogenous chemicals (cannabinoids, opioids) while others, such as the hallucinogens, interfere with communication between parts of the brain, producing changes in perception and the attribution of meaning. These are very significant differences between drugs. Drugs are also understood to vary in other important ways, such as in the difference between opioids and stimulants in producing physical dependence and a withdrawal syndrome. The literature analysed here is far less consistent in its recognition of the variations between drugs; indeed, its desire to compare and contrast overeating and obesity with 'drug addiction' regularly produces generalising statements about drugs. For example, in making a case for the links between overeating and addiction, Pelchat observes:

> A study of neurochemistry of reward provides a great deal of evidence for similarity between food and drug cravings... Drug abuse is

associated with decreased sensitivity of the dopamine-reward system. The same is true in obese individuals. (2009, 621)

Similarly, in the abstract to their article on the evidence for food addiction, Liu et al. (2010, 133) explain that '[g]ood or great smelling, looking and tasting food has characteristics similar to that of drugs of abuse'. The authors go on to posit sugar as an addictive substance, citing its capacity to cause the release of endogenous opioids and dopamine in the brain as the basis for its classification as addictive. This classification is backed up by the assertion that sugar consumption 'follows the typical addiction pathway that consists of bingeing, withdrawal, craving, and cross-sensitisation' (2010, 134).

Ifland et al. (2009) also frame foods as potential drugs in their own right, targeting 'refined food' with high levels of salt, sugar, refined carbohydrates, fat and caffeine as potentially addictive. Overconsumption of drugs, they argue, follows 'the very same mechanisms – pleasure seeking followed by mindless behavioural reinforcement – that are operative in the loss of control over certain foods' (2009, 519). As described in the previous section on addiction, comparative statements of this kind enact addiction as defined by a set of fixed attributes, even when some, such as withdrawal, are not considered in the addiction field to apply consistently across drugs. Similarly, 'drugs' operate as a useful comparator for 'food', coalescing as a unitary reality even as neuroscience seeks to distinguish the effects on brain chemistry of different drugs. Beyond this homogenisation of 'drugs', the category is also subjected to expansion by proposals to include particular foods as drugs. Sugar or 'refined' food's effect on the brain is key to its reclassification, as are other putative effects such as bingeing and withdrawal. If sugar is to become a drug, what are drugs to become? The category of drugs must surely break down or change if everyday substances such as sugar are introduced.

Of course, while we would not wish to draw a clear line between food and drugs given the latter is, as already argued, a purely political category, there are differences of some significance between the two categories as they are conventionally understood. The most obvious of these is that substances conventionally categorised as drugs – cocaine, heroin, alcohol, nicotine and so on – are not necessary for life. Food, as already noted, certainly is, and while it is possible to abstain from cocaine, heroin and alcohol, it is not possible to abstain from food. This has implications for the way addiction is conceived. It must allow room to move in the cramped conceptual territory on which the inconvenient dilemma, 'food is good/food is bad', is emerging in this field.

Much discussion of obesity or 'food addiction' addresses this dilemma by openly or implicitly distinguishing between need and want, a distinction that is not necessary to notions of drug addiction in that the body has no physiological 'need' for drugs, and distinctions between healthy, essential levels of consumption and unhealthy, excessive levels of consumption do not make sense.

The scientific literature varies in its response to this issue of need and want. Much of the research draws on a newly created category of food, mentioned above, sometimes termed 'refined', sometimes 'highly palatable' food. These terms refer to foods high in sugar and/or fat and/or salt, and most often, again explicitly or by implication, cheap 'junk' food. As we saw in the case of sugar, this focus works to produce some foods as drugs, juxtaposing them against healthy or natural foods, in that they are excessively dense in flavour and energy, and therefore like drugs in their chemistry, able to overstimulate the brain. As with other drugs, this overstimulation creates a feedback loop of reward and withdrawal that produces, or in itself constitutes, an addictive state. Here, the problem of food as an intrinsically healthy, essential aspect of life is overcome by creating a limited category of non-essential drug-like foods. It is this group of foods that, for some (such as Volkow & Wise 2005), should be consumed only at low levels, or, for others (such as Ifland et al. 2009), is so drug-like, so ready to alter brain chemistry and cause addiction, that it should be avoided altogether. A notable exception to this approach is that of Rogers and Smit (2000) who, relatively early in the rise of the neuroaddiction model of obesity, argue that any food can become addictive if it is administered according to the right patterns of constraint and bingeing. Addiction is, in this article, made more by denial than by excess. It is difficult to ignore the reference to financial support from the enticingly named Biscuit, Cake, Chocolate and Confectionery Alliance, London, in the conflict of interest disclosure that concludes this article, but to make too much of this apparent conflict would be to treat other science as purer and more disinterested than an STS approach such as ours would allow.

A second approach to the problem of food as drug is to locate the origins of addiction not primarily in the character of the particular food but in the structure of the brain itself, and to distinguish between more susceptible brains and less susceptible brains. Susceptibility comes in more than one form however. As Davis et al. explain:

> Low opioid signalling [in some brains] could foster overeating (and drug use) in some individuals as a form of 'self-medication', while

in others, enhanced opioid signalling could promote greater intake of palatable food (and drug use) because of the heightened pleasure experienced from these substances. (2011, 1352)

Both this approach and the approach that treats some foods as intrinsically addictive see brain function as a set of mechanisms able to produce addiction. The latter differs from the former, however, in placing the main emphasis on the brain's built-in vulnerability to addiction, presenting food of any kind as potentially addictive when it is consumed under particular circumstances – that is, if it is associated with a reward.

These two approaches will not be new to scholars of addiction. Despite their grounding in the relatively novel field of addiction neuroscience, they reproduce a familiar debate about the origins of drug addiction: is addiction caused by characteristics of the drug, or is it the product of an internal flaw in the addicted individual? In responding to drug addiction, in attempting to reduce its incidence, should we focus on individuals and their vulnerabilities or on drugs and their intrinsically toxic or corrupting properties? Should we seek to reduce supply of the corrupting drug or demand from vulnerable individuals? Of course, Western liberal democracies have tended to do both, placing individuals into disease categories and identifying factors that lead to individual vulnerability to addiction, while also attempting to limit access to (at least some) drugs in the belief that such drugs have their own destiny, able to corrupt whomever they come into contact with. Vociferous debate accompanies the changes in emphasis that shift over time between these approaches, yet, again, this knowledge-making process of debate is washed away in this literature's enactments of addiction.

Obesogenics: Making 'environment'

Implicit in the issues covered in the preceding sections is the preoccupation in the scientific literature with two actors: the body and the substance. In much of this material, the substance acts on the body and the body acts on the substance. Downplayed, even absent, is any recognisable notion of the social in shaping or informing this most social of practices, eating. This is not the case for all health-related approaches to eating and obesity, which encompass perspectives from public health, geography and anthropology, among other disciplines, although, as indicated at the outset, critics have argued that many of these proposed solutions to obesity tend to oversimplify social, environmental and cultural factors (recommending individuals take more exercise and decrying 'obesogenic environments', for example, while ignoring the complex meanings and pleasures of food and eating). Even more limited in scope and intention, however, are efforts to incorporate social or environmental factors in the scientific literature explored here. As has been demonstrated, where obesity is enacted as an addiction, it has become subject to the recent shift in emphasis in addiction concepts to those of neuroscience. In the process, as we will see, any meaningful concept of the social is effectively silenced or ignored. There are many ways in which this occurs, and here we focus on one common textual practice: brief acknowledgment of the complexity of factors shaping eating and body size followed by the relegation of such factors to the periphery of the text, or indeed to silence – or deletion as Law (2011) might put it. We do not focus on this textual practice because we consider it unique to the field of obesity neuroscience. As we have seen in the chapters on research discourses of methamphetamine and alcohol, it is common to the neuroscience of drug addiction as well. Nevertheless, the neglect of the social has especial salience for this context in that food is widely embraced as a profoundly positive foundational social object, and lifting it out of its sociality has specific implications and effects.

How does this textual practice play out? A list of factors 'shaping' or 'influencing' overeating is often given in the abstract or opening paragraph of an article, with those factors closest to capturing the social ranked secondary to neuropsychological factors. Myslobodsky (2003, 121), for example, sets out to challenge the privileging of 'traditional environmental factors and lifestyle changes' in understanding overweight and obesity, arguing that 'the neuropsychiatric experience might be the most fundamental'. The concluding summary clarifies this further by supporting the notion of 'stimulus-bound behaviours'. These treat environmental causes as 'secondary to the internal state of the organism' (2003, 128). Following Law, we can see how the specific methodological demands of the knowledge-making processes employed here shape the concepts deployed and the conclusions Myslobodsky (2003, 127) draws: 'The utility of this "reductionist" mode of thinking in obesity research might be felt in de-emphasising the importance of multiple weak risk factors.'

NIDA Director Nora Volkow and her co-author Roy Wise (2005) make a rather different argument based on a similar, equally reductive, ranking strategy. They advocate the application of the idea of drug addiction to overeating, citing high-fat, high-calorie foods as the correlate for drugs of addiction and noting that 'exposure to powerful reinforcers' (2005, 555) is linked to the development of addiction to food and thus obesity. We read this notion of 'exposure' as the authors' initial formulation of the role of environment, or the social, in obesity. It is not, however, the primary factor in the problem. Instead, '[a]s much as 40–60% of the vulnerability to addiction and 50–70% of the variability in body mass index might be attributed to genetic differences' (2005, 555). The article goes on to review other contributors to obesity, following an opening section on genetics with a section on environmental factors. This category largely comprises junk food vending machines and fast-food restaurants. 'Stress' is also included, although this is characterised largely in terms of brain chemistry. Developmental factors follow environment. Here drug experimentation in adolescence is presented as a correlate for early exposure to problematic diets in utero and early life. 'Neurobiological mechanisms' (or the brain chemistry of eating) are then compared with those of drug use. The authors go on to a section on 'Neurobiological adaptations', arguing (in keeping with our findings in the previous section on the stabilisation of 'drugs' in this literature):

> The regulation of food consumption is much more complex than that of drug consumption because food intake is modulated by multiple peripheral and central signs, whereas drugs are modulated mostly by the drug's central effects. (2005, 557)

Here food consumption is necessarily more complex than drug consumption, which has little or no meaning beyond its 'central effects'. This comment clearly refers to more and less complex modulations in the brain, but we read it as also evacuating food consumption of social, personal and cultural meaning. Food consumption is endowed with more complexity than drug consumption, but its meaning and effects remain almost entirely accounted for by brain chemistry. This reductive treatment of socially and culturally produced individuals and their eating preferences and practices is prefigured in an earlier (unintentionally rather comical) construction that reads more like one of the literature's quite common accounts of laboratory rats. Drawing parallels between drug addiction and obesity, it describes both as the result of 'foraging and ingestion habits that persist and strengthen despite the threat of catastrophic consequences' (Volkow & Wise 2005, 555). When human beings 'forage' and 'ingest', they are surely confined to an extremely crudely understood social and cultural environment.

Other articles repeat this tendency to gesture towards, then wash away, the social. In some, social factors such as the ready availability of palatable food, modern sedentary lifestyle and economic issues (Carnell et al. 2011; Ifland et al. 2009) are cited only to be dismissed outright as contributory reasons for why humans overeat when they do not want to. As Ifland et al. put it:

> While some or all of these ideas may have some degree of explanatory power, none of them address a critical question; namely, why do people in industrial societies persistently overeat despite considerable repeated efforts not to do so? (2009, 524)

This article goes on to describe sugar, refined carbohydrates (such as flour), fat and salt as 'addictive substances', implying that this diagnosis is self-evidently more persuasive than the other factors cited. In concluding, the authors propose that '[i]n the absence of an addiction framework, irrational overeating of refined foods remains a puzzle without a solution' (2009, 524). Is eating highly palatable food in large quantities really so puzzling? Given that much of such eating occurs in positive contexts, such as meals among friends and family, at times with a significant sense of occasion, or in challenging contexts such as stressful or tedious work environments, and consistently with very indirect and complex (at best incremental) links to negative consequences, regular overeating with its attendant pleasures and compensations appears at very least unsurprising. In such cases, scientific explanations seem, in their thin, selective enactments of the social aspects of eating as 'environment', inadequate to the point of counter productive.

Fixing the body

Numerous other arresting collateral realities are produced in this literature, so many that a book on this topic alone would not exhaust them. The last one we explore here is that of the body, selected as it relates closely to those already discussed. As we will demonstrate, the obese body is enacted in both subtle and explicit ways as stable and self-evident in the literature. One of the most obvious ways this occurs is through the many comparisons that are drawn between obese persons and persons of a 'healthy' weight. Several articles describe experiments conducted on obese and slim individuals, the purpose of which is to identify differences in brain structure between the two, and hypothesise these differences as either causes or effects of obesity. Where this line of investigation is pursued, particular textual strategies are necessary to establish and maintain coherence; for example, cross-sectional or snapshot approaches to body size are used, such that individuals classifiable as obese or slim at the time of the research are treated as always already obese or slim, with any variation in body size over the life course hidden. Perhaps the most striking example of this can be found in Carnell et al.'s (2011) review of neuroimaging and obesity. The review reports on a range of studies comparing 'lean and obese adults' (2011, 45), finding significant differences between the two groups in cognition and brain structure. Some research, they report, 'demonstrated a linear association between higher BMI and smaller brain volume, particularly within the grey matter' (2011, 47). Obese people have, it seems, smaller brains. Several observations can be made about these statements, one being that the collateral realities they enact about obese people are unlikely to be well received by them, and indeed, look rather like the stigmatising generalisations once made about women or black people, now debunked and seen as all too obviously based in prejudice. For the purposes of this chapter, however, our more general point is that the research enacts obese and lean individuals as mutually exclusive categories, that is, obesity and leanness as permanent states such that statements about other intrinsic bodily differences are considered viable. In short, such research treats body size as fixed, implying that the fat have always been and will always be fat, and likewise the slim. Of course, if we are to take feminists' observations about stigma associated with fat bodies seriously, essentialising body size in this way has significant social and political implications. Fat persons are different from slim persons (despite what is known about dieting, which tells us that bodies very often shift categories from fat to slim or back again). Obesity is essential to bodies and, where the brain is implicated, to subjects – a permanent, intrinsic weakness or flaw in the organism. While Carnell et al. (2011) admit that the research is not yet developed enough to distinguish causal direction (do smaller brains cause obesity or are they an effect of it?), they leave the fluidity of body size and its implications for such generalisations unexplored.

This enactment of the body as stable also occurs in other ways, for example, via stabilisations of the brain, its structure and its functions. We see this in work that suggests that obesity is caused either by underactive brain reward systems or, alternatively, overactive brain reward systems. Yet, as we have seen in previous chapters, the neuroscience of addiction also explicitly requires a view of the brain as changeable (or 'plastic'). This too is found in the obesity literature, in the material that conceives some foods as drugs and the brain as changed by consumption of these concentrated, drug-like foods. Is the brain fixed or is it plastic?

This question has particular salience for drugs and drug-like substances. The brain must be plastic if drugs are to be able to hijack the reward system and alter the body and the mind sufficiently to cause addiction. In this context the brain is highly plastic: vulnerable to change within a very short time frame and with relatively little prompting. Indeed, the vivid metaphor of the 'trigger' is often used to describe this swift process (see, for example, Miller et al. 2010; Carnell et al. 2011). Yet once addiction is underway, the brain is, it seems, intensely resistant to change. The brain is now hardly plastic. The groove in which it is stuck, worn by a few occasions of consumption, will now take years, decades, if ever, to be changed by other influences, other experiences.

This apparent contradiction is, as Law might put it, necessary for the institutional survival of the neuroscientific approach to addiction. Accounting for it tends to occur by reference to the exceptional intensity of drugs. Their unnatural chemistry means the brain has no evolved capacity to protect itself from them, and once addiction has set in, no access to non-drug experiences of sufficient intensity to disrupt the vicious cycle of overwhelming reward and withdrawal. Can food really stand in for drugs here? Again, this account relies on a novel drug-like category: highly palatable food, ranked above other food as more appealing, more satisfying and thus more dangerous, and the brain as just as susceptible to the body's intrinsic (evolved) preference for such foods as for drugs. In creating this category, the brain and body can be enacted as the same brain and body hijacked by, say, heroin or crystal meth. In this way, the body and the brain are stabilised to suit the enactment of overeating as a problem of addiction.

Conclusion

In this discussion of the scientific literature on obesity as addiction we identified four key collateral realities: addiction, drugs, environment and the body. Having done so, we must consider the way these four work together, enacting the neuroaddiction account of obesity as coherent. This is important because, as we have already said, this scientific discourse is likely to shape responses in the future. It is also important in what it means for addiction more broadly, for the notion and substance of drugs, and the contemporary (always already social) body. While obesity will be changed forever by these realities, our focus in this chapter has also been on how addiction too will be changed. Perhaps our most important conclusion on this count is to do with the tendency within this scientific literature to treat expertise on drug addiction as far more settled, consensual and effective than most of those working in that domain would consider accurate. If the obesity literature is to be believed, addiction is a thoroughly understood, well-integrated diagnosis for which there are a range of highly effective treatments. Drugs can sensibly be understood as a coherent category, and their effects generalised across individuals and social and cultural contexts. The bodies in which drugs work are predictable. The social world sometimes impacts on the problem of addiction, exacerbating it, but it is never seen as the source of the very norms and ideals from which anxieties about dependence emerge and gain meaning (Sedgwick 1993). If obesity experts take up drug addiction expertise, the obesity epidemic will be solved. Familiar strategies of supply reduction (regulation of highly palatable foods) and demand reduction (pharmaceutical interventions in brain chemistry) will do this work.

In some respects the meaning-making process around overeating, obesity and addiction neuroscience is circular. It is hardly surprising that, when drug addiction is understood as a malfunction of normal reward systems that govern eating (among other processes), eating comes to be open to addiction discourse. Here is one way of beginning to answer the question most forcefully raised by these accounts: how and why have cultures that produced such profoundly meaningful stories of food and eating as the Last Supper of the Christian tradition, and such highly refined eating practices as molecular gastronomy and the death-row prisoner's last meal, also begun to produce such constrained understandings of the meaning and symbolism of food and eating? Yet the effects of this process of meaning making, reality enactment, are more than circular. While they do produce important feedback loops of authorisation, such as the re-enactment of addiction as self-evident, and drug treatment as unquestionably effective, they enact new collateral realities too. The body is stabilised, as is the brain and by implication the subject. The relationship between the individual and the social is narrowed; indeed, as the social is reduced to 'environment', that most social of practices, eating is (perhaps paradoxically) enacted at times as less socially produced than drug consumption. Together, the four collateral realities support and authorise each other. Uniform drugs cause clear cases of addiction in fixed bodies. All this occurs within a simple, secondary environment. Made this way, the reality of food addiction offers itself to science for correction. Drugs can be identified and controlled. Addicts can be diagnosed and treated. Obesogenic environments can be regulated. Bodies can be restored. Amid the unknowns can be found some certainties it seems. Having identified this striking note of certainty within the many questions left to modern obesity science, we next find ourselves asking how closely these certainties align with lay articulations of overeating and obesity. To what extent do we see the realities of food addiction enacted in the scientific literature also 'done' in public accounts of food, eating and obesity? How well, that is, do the realities enacted within neuroscience hold together beyond the specific authorising context in which they emerged? In the next chapter we explore public accounts of these phenomena, asking how closely expert and public realities align.

7
Stepping to the Side of Addiction: Everyday Realities of Overeating and Obesity

Having explored in Chapter 6 the collateral realities being made in scientific literature on overeating and obesity, we next track these collateral realities – addiction, drugs, the social (or environment) and the body – into public accounts to see how closely the two align. Our aim here is to identify the commonalities and differences between the two discursive domains, speculating on where, and how effectively, the scientific approach is holding together. As we have maintained throughout this book, whether a certain reality holds together depends on practice (Law 2011). How much coherence is enacted between scientific and public accounts? How much of the scientific reality of food addiction currently being made within science is practised in wider discourse? How much coherence exists at this time?

In answering these questions, this chapter draws on 30 interviews conducted with women in Melbourne, Australia. These interviews formed part of a study exploring mothers' and childcare workers' engagements with, and responses to, childhood obesity prevention education (see the Appendix for more details about data collection methods). In discussing these issues, however, almost all the participants referred in detail to their own experiences of food, eating and body weight, and in the process of discussing these issues we explored questions of compulsive eating and 'food addiction'. As we will find, while the brain science account of food addiction is coming to be accepted in scientific discourse, it is yet to dominate public discourse. Indeed, the interviews take a far more prosaic, and in some respects nuanced, view of eating than does the science. Mostly untouched by neuroscience, they consistently cite subtle social, emotional and cultural factors in accounting for individual eating patterns and food consumption in general. Such explanations offer flexibility in explaining weight gain and loss, in identifying variation both between individuals and within the individual over time. In these accounts, what science might call addiction is enacted as a habituated response to social and emotional processes in which the meaning of food is seen to build and change social relationships and alter individual experiences of daily life. Addiction is not ruled out here in explaining obesity; yet in these accounts of food, daily life and pleasure, far more expansive realities are enacted. In reaching these conclusions, we will speculate on the future of food addiction and, in turn, addiction in general.

We begin by analysing the participants' statements about food, obesity and addiction. In the section that follows we consider the participants' statements on the relationship between food and drugs, and the idea that food might act as a drug. The last two sections consider the place of the social and the body in women's discussions of food and eating.

The trickiness of addiction

In Chapter 6 we noted that the scientific literature framing overeating and obesity as addiction disorders draws on the *DSM* criteria for addiction (or 'dependence') and other classifying tools (such as the WHO definition) to compare features of eating with those of drug consumption. We argued that this literature tends to take for granted definitions of addiction, in some places selecting particular criteria as common to both overeating and drug use, in others juxtaposing overeating with drug use as a means of preserving eating as normal and distinguishing natural (healthy) foods from unnatural (addictive) foods and so on. In the process, statements asserting the similarity of overeating to 'drug addiction' are made, with 'drug addiction' enacted as stable, self-evident and unitary. Because the interviews we conducted almost exclusively involved women without any formal training in psychology, physiology or any other discipline currently engaged in knowledge making about obesity, the accounts they offer of addiction draw no such specific comparisons (although two participants with direct professional experience of contemporary public health and psychological research on addiction come much closer to the realities enacted in the previous section than do the 28 other participants). At the same time, some features of the formal definitions appear regularly in these accounts, the emphasis often falling, in the case of food, on the same features as it did in scientific accounts, in particular, on craving rather than repetition. Almost all participants agreed that food can be addictive, and that overeating is probably a form of addiction. Yet these apparent coherences with the scientific literature need to be read carefully, especially because the criteria on which women base their assessments often differ in tone and implication even as they broadly resemble those used in the scientific accounts.

Overall, the most common features of addiction cited by participants when discussing food addiction and asked what they mean by 'addiction' are those to do with craving, compulsion or urges, and dependence, need and the idea that the addict 'can't do without' the substance in question. Yet women's definitions are hard to sum up, and attempting to do so can erase their most salient quality – that of multiplicity and inconsistency. Caroline (aged 42), for example, defines addiction in this way:

> Oh, addiction is something that you can't give up, literally that you can't give up. I know because my husband and I were smokers [...] we haven't smoked since I was pregnant. I gave up before we started trying – yes, something that you can't give up that is constantly like... it's like a train of thought really, you know. But I also think it's a habit because now, like we don't smoke at all because we don't have that habit [...] but I think once you get into a habit of a certain way that's how it is and you don't know any better. So yes, I think habit and addiction go together personally.

Caroline's account captures one of the most taxing questions of addiction research and treatment, a question we formulated in the previous chapter in terms of brain plasticity in the neuroscientific model but which has taken a range of forms over time: if addiction means one is unable to cease consumption, how is it that so many seen as and self-identified as addicts do cease consumption? (Keane 2002). As Caroline puts it, struggling to achieve coherence, addiction is 'something that you can't give up, literally that you can't give up. I know because my husband and I were smokers [...] we haven't smoked since I was pregnant. I gave up before we started trying'. Inability to cease is articulated via cessation. In this respect Caroline's account reflects the incoherence and instability of addiction itself. Our point is not that she directly challenges accounts that take the stability of addiction for granted, rather that her account cannot hold together with the confidence found in the scientific literature. This ambiguity is common in the interviews, often accompanied by more explicitly expressed ambivalence.

Later Caroline is asked whether she sees food as an addictive substance, and she replies that the two are both the same and different:

> I think it's the same. I think it's like alcohol, tobacco, drugs, you know, I don't know, cocaine or whatever. Yes, I think it's the same. It's the same addiction but a different type I guess. Like, the actual thing you're taking is different, and they can kill you, so it's the same to me.

Magda (35) also offers an ambivalent take on addiction. Discussing overeating, she says:

> I don't know, I guess it could be an addiction as much as anything else could be an addiction, because you get addictions from things that are good, things that make you feel good [...] You take drugs because they feel good. If they feel good you want to do it more, and the more you do it the more you want it, the more you need it to feel good.

When asked what she means by addiction, Magda replies:

> Something that you feel you need, that you can't live without. Well, in saying that, I'm addicted to smoking but I know I can live without it [...] so yeah, I don't know, that's a tricky one to explain. Addiction is something you don't have the willpower to stop, I suppose. Maybe that's a better way to explain it. Even though I know smoking is bad for me [...] I still smoke. So that doesn't make sense at all, you know what I mean, so it's an addiction [...] And with food, a lot of people lack the willpower to say no. I know if something is really delicious and I'm full I might keep eating it because it's really delicious. I'm not addicted to it, but I should be able to stop when I'm full.

Is Magda addicted to the delicious food she describes or not? Yes and no. Willpower, or its absence, is a key feature of addiction, but when it comes to food, it both does and does not mean addiction. Dependence is important: the sense that you can't live without something. But the knowledge that you can may be present too. Fundamentally, addiction occurs with those things that make you feel good. In this sense Magda echoes, if not in the same terms, the core neuroscientific feature of addiction – its engagement with reward or 'feeling good'.

Beyond this, however, Magda's account, like Caroline's, departs significantly from the coherence enacted in scientific discourse. Addiction is not simple – instead it is 'tricky'. While some might be tempted to explain these ambiguous enactments of addiction as the effect of a lesser degree of formal knowledge than is available to the scientists publishing on food addiction, this would belie the acknowledgment in the broader scientific, social science and psychological literature that addiction is indeed a slippery, mutable concept and state (Keane 2002). Likewise, while some of the ambiguity likely emerges from the uncertain position into which this discourse places food – as necessary but indulgent, health-giving but potentially toxic – these extracts do not rely on food alone. Tellingly, they also cite smoking, hinting perhaps at where food most meaningfully fits in lay understandings of addiction. Like smoking, eating is normal rather than marginal. Although smoking has in recent decades become seen as unhealthy, smokers are not denigrated as 'addicts' in the classic sense – as decadent or broken subjects, dysfunctional, corrupting and untrustworthy.

Almost every participant interviewed on the nature of addiction offered multiple, internally inconsistent responses characterised by statements of confusion and uncertainty, especially when the question of food as potentially addictive was addressed. Does addiction rely on pleasure or not? Does it really mean one cannot stop? Must it involve something that is 'bad for you'? If a substance or activity is harmful, does this mean addiction is definitely present? Is craving in the mind or the body, or both? Is the mind the same as the brain? Following John Law's invitation to analyse the production of collateral realities, we can say that within public discourse on obesity, addiction is enacted as multiple and confusing, 'tricky' and difficult to pin down. It is a real problem but, especially where food is implicated, an elusive and confusing one.

Beyond this inability or refusal to make addiction cohere in discussions of overeating and obesity, the interviews depart from the scientific accounts in another significant way. In the context of food, addiction is explained using terms that approximate key features of conventional addiction concepts, but in a mode that downplays pathologisation and instead imparts a sense of the common sense drivers and pleasures of overeating. Here we are thinking in particular of the concept of 'habit'.

Caroline has already introduced the idea of habit into her understanding of addiction:

> I also think it's a habit because now like we don't smoke at all because we don't have that habit [...] but I think once you get into a habit of

> a certain way that's how it is and you don't know any better. So yes, I think habit and addiction go together personally.

Is habit addiction, or does it simply accompany addiction? Caroline is not clear on this – instead of specifying the nature of addiction, the word is given a different role, which is to render addiction in commonplace, relatively harmless terms. Habits are, as we discussed in the Introduction to this book, as helpful as they are harmful. To recap, the *Oxford English Dictionary* (online version accessed on 8 July 2013) defines it as '1a: settled or regular tendency or practice, especially one that is hard to give up'. While repetition is not always conceived positively, especially in relation to drugs (Fraser & valentine 2008), it is hard to dispute the gentler overtones of 'habit' as compared to 'addiction'. Ella (26) also refers to habit in trying to explain addiction:

> I don't know, a lot of it is habit as well I guess. Addiction, I don't know, like I don't know, you can't stop doing what you're doing, I guess, or your mind is telling you that you can't.

As with Caroline, the link between the two is left vague; indeed, Ella's main emphasis here seems to be on her sense that she 'doesn't know'. Glenda's use of the idea of habit is rather more specific:

> Yeah I don't know whether it's food, the actual food as such that would be the addiction or, I don't know... or the fact of just eating, that habit and maybe that's what drives that addiction, if I am making sort of sense. I'm thinking that some food can be addictive, sugar and caffeine, that kind of stuff probably could be addictive for people, but I think it's more than just the food, I think it's, I think it's a behavioural kind of thing as well, so that would be more psychological kind of too... because it's more about the behaviour than the actual food as such, maybe more of a habit or something, there is some kind of link to why it's food and not something else.

While Glenda (aged 32) does not explicitly distinguish foods from conventional drugs (indeed she considers sugar and, perhaps less surprisingly, caffeine as drugs), she uses habit to create a category in which repetition and the effect of this on the psyche create its own force. Here, it is not the food per se that is addictive, but the act of repetition involved in consuming the food. In doing so, Glenda leaves untouched the question of why this food is consumed repetitively, and does not spell out whether she is thinking of all foods (aside from sugar and caffeine) here, or particular ones. Helen (46) too is uninclined to ascribe an unqualified notion of addiction to food, drawing, like Glenda, on the idea of habit. When asked if she considers overeating to be an addiction, she says: 'Probably not so much an addiction as a habit.'

While Caroline and Glenda seem to deploy habit as a means of avoiding the harsher implications of 'addiction', however, Helen's goal turns out to be rather different. Pressed to define addiction, she says:

> It's actually a bit of a tough one for me. My brother-in-law is an alcoholic which has actually caused the breakdown of his marriage and separation from his child and, you know, he says he is addicted to alcohol and he can't change, and I have a really hard time... if you've got a little boy who is four, how can you not bloody change for him, do you know what I mean? [...] I haven't been in that position – I don't think I have ever been addicted to anything or felt that strongly about something that I can't stop for whatever reason, so I would presume that would be my answer for an addiction, something that you just can't, again I'm sort of a bit, it's not 'can't', it's 'won't' – won't change.

While for some habit offers a means of characterising compulsion to eat in terms less judgemental than those offered by addiction, for Helen 'addiction' represents an unwarranted escape from responsibility and thus judgement. 'Habit' refers to a choice for which one can be held responsible, whether this relates to eating or to more explicitly damaging consumption (as with alcohol). So when asked to clarify whether for her food is like other addictive substances, her reply emphasises agency rather than compulsion: 'Well, I suppose it's the same if you wanted to make that choice.' Significantly, Helen describes never having had a personal experience of compulsive feelings.

Petra (aged between 35 and 40) too shows a reluctance to ascribe addiction to overeating, suggesting that laziness, depression, effort and motivation all contribute to obesity:

> It sounds horrible to say that they're lazy, but it's not just lazy, I think it's depression as well, and I know what it's like to be in a bigger body

> and feel like crap. It takes a lot of effort sometimes to push yourself to [change], you know, it does, and I can imagine living like that for a long time. It's become routine, it's habit, it's addictive.

Like Helen, Petra uses habit to deprive the obese of the exculpatory power of addiction. In this respect both exemplify and lend weight to Davis and Carter's (2009) assertion that addiction offers the obese an escape from notions of failure. The great majority of references to habit made in the interviews were, however, much more in keeping with Caroline and Glenda's. Would Helen and Petra change their apparently rather intolerant views of obesity if exposed to the neuroscience discourse of food addiction? Could 'doing' this addiction reality alleviate fat stigma, as neuroscientists often claim is the advantage of their approach? Public contact with obesity neuroscience is of course in its infancy, as is the field itself – that is, this addiction reality does not yet hold together very well beyond the scientific literature – so this remains to be seen. If obesity neuroscience's enactment of drug addiction is any guide, however, its potential to alleviate fat stigma is likely to be small. Likewise, if we are to take seriously the insights offered by social scientists and feminists about the profoundly entrenched abjection of fat, femininity and dependence at the heart of neo-liberal modernity, a turn to disease models and their attendant stigmas of dependence and 'invalidity' hardly promise radical change.

Not for the first time in this book, we turn to Eve Sedgwick's (1993) classic critique of addiction attribution, and her formulation of habit, which she sees as offering an 'otherwise' to addiction attribution. As we have already argued, this idea is

> not opposed to [addiction] or explanatory of it, but rather one step to the side of it [...] a version of repeated action that moves, not towards metaphysical absolutes [of absolute voluntarity or absolute compulsion], but toward interrelations of the action – and the self acting. (1993, 138)

Of course, as we have also noted, Sedgwick warns us that this notion still requires a great deal of work if it is to 'sidestep' 'the twin hurricanes named Just Do It and Just Say No' offered to subjects of contemporary neo-liberalism. Still, Sedgwick sees potential in habit's promise of something conceptually better than addiction, and it seems that many of our participants agree. If overeating is, for many, a kind of habit, familiar but tricky, addiction yet not addiction, is food seen as the same as drugs? As we found in Chapter 6, neuroscience is progressively enacting the two as the same, but what of the public realities of addiction?

Food and drugs: Like and unlike

Almost all our interview participants endorsed the idea that food acts like a drug – or is a drug. As Anna (30) explains:

> I think addiction is just liking something and just doing the same thing you know. Whether it's good or bad and whether you're full or so... I think addiction is the same, whether it's food or other substances.

Caroline, too, explicitly associates the two:

> I think it's the same. I think it's like alcohol, like tobacco, drugs, you know, I don't know, cocaine or whatever, yes, I think it's the same. It's the same addiction but a different type I guess, like the actual thing that you're taking is different [but] they can all kill you so it's the same to me.

Leah (38) presents the most comprehensive picture of the links between food and other addictive substances. Her professional background produces a distinctive account that takes in three main factors, emotional addiction to food, the neurochemical effects of refined foods and genetics (her comments are worth quoting at length):

> [It depends how you define addiction]. I think you can have emotional addictions in that people don't feel control over their behaviour – behaviour that they want to stop but they feel they can't. If that's what an addiction is then certainly obesity can be an addiction. If it's a physiological thing, if it's something that is, is physiologically driven [...] I think a lot of processed foods have ingredients that do just mess around with our normal body's homeostasis, and my first degree is in neuroscience and I study [...] the mechanisms on a neuroscientific basis that relate to these things and yeah, that's why I stay away from processed food as much as possible [...] I just think it messes on a neuroscientific, you know, on a synaptic level often with certain signals. So yeah, I have no doubt that there is a physiological component for some people [...] I think they

> [some processed foods] do induce people to eat more than is, for their sensations of hunger, physical hunger, that maybe are misleading.

Having identified emotional and neurochemical causes of obesity, Leah also refers to genetic causes:

> But I think the majority, the reason most people are obese is probably because I think there's just a strong genetic component that isn't an addictive issue, some people are just bigger.

Among those who identify similarities between food and drugs, some add caveats, expressing ambivalence about including food in that category. Several, for example, argue for the need to distinguish between food's necessary role in health and the absence of any such role for drugs. Wendy (35) explains:

> I think overeating is an addiction and I think it comes from, well, it's like some people drink, some people take drugs, but with food I think it's on another level because we need food to live, do you know what I mean? It's not like taking away the cigarettes and the alcohol, so yeah [...] I think it comes from, some people would call it emotional eating, yeah.

Here, food is both like and unlike other addictive substances: its necessary place in life and its links to the emotions mean it cannot be seen as just another drug. Colleen (63), too, emphasises the role of need in eating, but points to the line that must be drawn between necessary food and unnecessary overeating:

> You need to eat to make yourself survive, be fit, strong and healthy, you don't need to eat because its, you want to keep eating and eating and then you think, there's a problem there.

Like Colleen, Glenda identifies some links between food and other addictive substances, defining addiction as both physical and psychological.

> Yeah...I suppose the best way I can explain it is both a physical and psychological need for either food or whatever it is that you're addicted to I suppose, it can be both physical and psychological addiction.

Despite sharing many attributes, however, food and other addictive substances should not, in Glenda's view, be conflated:

> I don't know whether it's food, the actual food as such that would be the addiction or [...] the fact of just eating, that habit and maybe that's what drives that addiction, if I am making sort of sense. I'm thinking that some food can be addictive, sugar and caffeine, and that kind of stuff probably could be addictive for people but I think it's more than just the food, I think it's, I think it's a behavioural kind of thing as well, so that would be more psychological kind of too.

Here Glenda seems to argue that food addiction is more psychological than other addictions, that it is based on 'habit' rather than on the addictive properties of the food. When the interviewer attempts to clarify her view, this distinction is drawn more clearly:

> INTERVIEWER: Yeah right and I suppose there are other substances that might be more... create a physical dependency?
>
> GLENDA: Yes [...] because it's more about the behaviour than the actual food as such, maybe more of a habit or something, there is some kind of link to why it's food and not something else but yeah...

Unlike these participants, Marie, Michelle and Sarah all directly dispute the idea that food is an addictive substance, arguing that our legitimate physical need for it sets it apart:

> Look it's very different. Yes. I would say that no, you know I smoked for many years and still have the occasional one and I know there is a big difference. The major difference is that food is not a bad thing, it is a good thing for you, whereas you find most other addictive substances are not good for you in any... you can't justify them and sort of you know, they're not keeping you alive, it's a chemical treat I suppose, whereas food we actually do need to have. Food is actually something essential, so you kind of want to be addicted to it otherwise you know you would be dead. We're programmed to seek out food and you know, because obviously it's a biological necessity. So, yes, very different to other addictive substances which are not in any way necessary for life. Which just makes it so much sadder that you can't have as much as you want anyway. (Marie, 42)

Like Marie, Michelle (32) separates food from drugs by pointing to its essential role in life:

> It's, well, food is different because we all need food to survive. We all need to eat in some form, we can't give up eating. We can give up smoking, we can give up drinking, give up drugs and survive you can't give up eating so, yes, it's very different.

Michelle also makes another argument separating food from drugs, based on the pleasure of eating:

> And food, you know, food, like any other thing, food is very pleasurable, it's a big part of our life and we need it to survive. It is very different.

Here Michelle's argument seems to have two strands. Food differs from drugs because it is not something we can give up or abstain from. It also differs from drugs because... but here her point is rather less clear. Food is pleasurable, yet so too, of course, are drugs. It could be that this reference to the pleasure of eating, and the follow-up remark that it is a big part of life, points to the more complex, elusive social and cultural role food plays, one which, by implication, the consumption of other substances does not entail.

The question of pleasure comes up in many of the interviews when compulsive eating or obesity is discussed. Some see the pleasure of food as the source of its addictive power – delicious foods are difficult to resist. But the role of pleasure in understanding why some people overeat is much less pronounced than in the scientific literature. While the neuroscience account stresses the brain-changing role of intense pleasure, relying heavily on this idea to explain its notion of food addiction, these accounts refer much more often to the more modest satisfactions of 'comfort eating'. As Petra puts it:

> [Y]our body might not be hungry but your mind needs it so you just sit there and eat and eat and eat and eat. Again, that can be depression as well, where you're comforting yourself, things have gone wrong in your life and you're feeling miserable, you feel better when you eat a bit of chocolate and you just keep eating it because it tastes good.

Pleasure and comfort eating are seen as contributing to overeating and obesity for many. Leah, on the other hand, makes a very different argument, quite at odds with the neuroscience account of eating, pleasure and brain chemistry on which she relies elsewhere in her interview. In most cases, taking pleasure in food, according to Leah, protects against overeating:

> If people really enjoy their food, I think conversely they're less likely to overeat, you know. Unless people are overeating from really a deep-seated emotional need for escape, you know, I think people are less likely to overeat really high quality food that they've really enjoyed. If they have a sense of genuine pleasure in what they eat then they say the pleasure has happened and they stop. If they're eating either lacklustre food or food that just isn't hitting the spot for whatever reason, of course they're going to keep on going and attempt to gain some sense of pleasure that ultimately may not arrive.

Hannah (aged between 35 and 40) is convinced neither of the dangers of food's pleasures nor of its protective effects. Instead, she is much less clear about the place of pleasure in overeating and addiction:

> HANNAH: I am addicted to drinking coffee but yeah, I think addiction is, yeah, something that you really need but usually it's negative things, either drugs or alcohol or tobacco. I wouldn't see eating as an addiction. In France we mainly speak about eating as a pleasure so culturally, for me, eating cannot be an addiction except in very specific medical problems.
>
> INTERVIEWER: So you associate addiction with things that aren't pleasurable?
>
> HANNAH: No, because actually I like drinking coffee, some people like, yeah, no, I don't know, I've never thought about this. Negative in terms of negative effects? Yeah. Tobacco is not good for health, so, but that might be a pleasure around smoking, so yeah, I don't know.

Across the interviews, then, significant differences can be found in the way food is understood as compared with the scientific literature, both in terms of the place it is given as a drug and also in terms of the meaning and role of pleasure in overeating and obesity. Some participants construct coherent accounts on these issues, but as in the previous section's discussion of addiction, many struggle to achieve and maintain coherence and certainty. The transcripts are replete with efforts to contrast or reconcile individual foods, individual drugs as like or not like each other in effects and implications: drinking coffee, smoking, eating chocolate, taking cocaine, indulging in sugar. While these strategies sometimes achieve a local coherence, with different notions of drugs enacted at different moments, viewed together the interviews do not suggest that the food addiction reality increasingly forcefully enacted in the scientific literature, in which foods are drugs and pleasure's ability to change the brain must be feared, is yet holding together beyond that technical context. As was found in the previous section, the complexity and ambivalence articulated in our interviews enact a much more layered and multiple series of realities.

Beyond 'environment'

How do the scientific enactments of the 'environment' of eating and obesity discussed in the previous chapter compare with those articulated in the women's interviews we consider here? As we argued in Chapter 6, the neuroscientific literature enacts the social context of food and eating exceedingly thinly. The 'obesogenic environment' causes individuals to eat too much highly processed and addictive food. As a result, their brains are corrupted; they gain weight and lose control over their consumption practices. How do our interview participants understand the context of food and eating? Interviewed about both their own eating habits and their children's, they draw a far richer picture of the meaning of food and overeating than does the scientific literature. Much of this emerges in conversations about their daily practices in feeding their children, encouraging healthy eating and taking part in the pleasure of eating. Celeste (35), for example, describes the pleasure she finds in shopping for food and then cooking it with her son:

> I sort of get excited about it. And I walk into the supermarket or the market and just go, 'I just wanna buy everything because I can create these amazing things with it.'

Also important is the context in which food is eaten. Celeste describes regular family meal rituals in which takeaway food or pizza plays an important role:

> We do like to have family meals. Quite often on a Friday we'll either make our own pizza or we'll get Indian take-away and we'll sit and have a Friday night picnic party. And we just get a blanket, and we'll

watch a movie or just sit and have a game, or whatever, and just eat together.

Similarly, Margaret (40) explains the role of 'junk' food in family socialising:

MARGARET: Yeah, like you know, chips [...] when you sit down to watch a movie, we will pull out something then. That's when the kids – I will say, 'come on, we'll watch a movie and we'll eat a packet of chips', or we'll eat our chocolate and our junk food when we're watching something.
INTERVIEWER: Yep and that's part of the enjoyment or the experience?
MARGARET: Yeah, that's it, but like I don't put honey or that on me food or anything, to make me kids eat it. I would rather them taste the actual vegetable rather than just hide it, if you know what I mean. That's why I don't let them stick sauce everywhere, because sauce is bad for you, isn't it?

Margaret is telling us that there are moments in which the ritual associated with food – here junk food, and not incidentally, but precisely because of its status as an indulgence – helps create a moment of family togetherness. This does not mean she neglects to consider health when preparing food for her family. As she explains, she prefers to introduce her children to the 'actual' taste of vegetables and avoids adding honey or (tomato) sauce to make the vegetables more palatable. The balance Margaret seeks between pleasures, health and family sociality is common among our participants, yet it is noticeably out of step with the neuroscientific literature which emphasises the corrupting power of junk food – the risk that exposure (even at modest levels) will change the brain and inaugurate a cycle of damaging addiction.

Some participants also emphasised the cultural significance of food. Hannah, a French-born participant, explains that for her eating is intrinsically social and that for the French it must be pleasurable and communal:

Yeah, for me it's very important and culturally in France it's very important. It's a pleasure and it's, yeah, eating is a pleasure and eating together is even more pleasure. You would not eat as often alone in France. It's a moment of sharing.

Similarly, Marie explains that her cultural background informs her approach to food and eating, characterised as it is by the communication of love:

> Look, with an Asian mother as well, I mean [...] food is a way of showing love and affection in a lot of cultures.

The social connections made possible by, or enhanced by, food also extend beyond the family and the special place food has in some cultures for the family. As Marie observes, different cultures introduce new cuisines, enriching life for everyone:

> Like, places like Victoria St [a predominantly Vietnamese dining precinct in Melbourne] are a testament to the fact that any palate can adjust and that food is real pleasure for so many people.

This openness to the pleasures of food can be seen, Marie argues, in the popularity of television programmes on food and cooking:

> There are so many programs on at the moment [about cooking] and it just shows you how many of us actually see it as one of the real pleasures in life.

Marie's comments point to a multifaceted role for food in daily life: it helps create and sustain family, it introduces and expresses cultural diversity, it entertains. In short, it is one of life's 'real' – elsewhere she pointedly says 'few' – pleasures.

Overall, our participants invest food with far more complex and powerful meanings, enact it as much more thoroughly social – as culturally and subjectively constitutive – than does the scientific literature. Indeed, the literature's invocations of the 'environment' in which eating occurs, with its references to fast-food outlets and supermarket junk foods, seem singularly poorly equipped to grasp the eating articulated here, including overeating or 'unhealthy' eating. In imposing the notion of addiction, it seems, this literature must reduce eating to a small group of rudimentary elements – foraging and feeding in one case. How will this gulf between the subjectivity and sociality of food and eating, and the scientific approach to it, be bridged? That the two need to be made to hold together better would seem key if the neuroscientific approach and the measures it promotes for avoiding obesity are to find a receptive audience. Yet a question remains as to whether a neuroaddiction model of overeating and obesity would survive a more thoroughgoing appreciation of the sociality of food. While our participants embrace both an addiction model of overeating and a social model of food, with one or two exceptions, they do not turn to brain chemistry to explain addiction. In this way, they leave much more room for the many elusive, ineffable, yet indispensable social and cultural elements of eating, and the benefits of overeating or eating junk food.

Balancing bodies

The last of the four collateral realities we identified in the scientific literature on obesity was that of the stable body, the body that does not change – in size or in the attributes or qualities that make it more or less disposed towards obesity. In the interview accounts of food, eating and obesity, no such body can be found. Some participants concur that obesity is a significant public health problem, but, rather like the interviewees we questioned about drinking, who were reluctant to generalise about alcohol addiction, the majority resist making blanket statements about overeating and fat and their impact on health. Instead, many exhibit impatience with public health messages that treat fat as pathological and the overweight as necessarily sick. As Holly (40) says, explaining her family's health:

> I feel that a lot of health is targeted at weight and I don't think weight is the only thing [...] You know, I am trying to eat healthy now so I don't have health problems in the future, and so I feel good and have energy now, and [yes] you want your weight to be reasonable because everyone wants to look good, let's face it [...] I want to have a good quality of life [...] but [too much is] about weight. So if you're the right weight then you don't have to worry about [health], and that's not true. You might have a fast metabolism but you could have shocking cholesterol or blood pressure or the whole heart disease. There are so many health issues.

Leah puts forward a similar view. Identifying a mismatch between public health knowledge about food and body size and individual experiences, she argues that public health has become oversimplifying and a source of unnecessary pressure:

> In relation to sort of buying into a wide-scale population level panic about obesity and policing that, to a degree I don't think it's helpful

> on an individual level [...] I just don't want my daughter being exposed to it too much. I want her to have a healthy, happy life and not be obsessing about what her weight is compared to her height. She'll know if she's, if we taught her as a child just to eat well and be responsive to her body's signal of hunger and fullness, and if she's doing that with decent, nutritious, whole foods I don't care how big or otherwise she is. You know, if her body type is, means that she's in the overweight category, if she's eating so that her body and soul and her mind are functioning and she's happy and healthy, I couldn't give a toss what her BMI [Body Mass Index] is [...] Her well-being is much more important to me than any increased risk of diabetes or whatever comes with obesity [...] It doesn't make any sense to me; it only makes people feel bad about themselves.

Both these comments enact a significant level of scepticism about current public health advice on body weight and health. This scepticism takes at least two forms: size does not necessarily determine healthiness, and health means more than physical health (it should encompass issues of well-being such as happiness and a 'functioning soul'). Leah and Holly are hardly alone in these views. Not only do other participants make similar points, but both issues are canvassed in depth in the critical social science literature on obesity discussed at the outset of the previous chapter.

A second way in which the body is framed differently in the interviews compared with the scientific literature is in the many ways it is at times treated as fluid and changing, rather than stable and monolithic. Youthful bodies, pregnant bodies, postnatal bodies, ageing bodies – some participants have experienced all these bodies, and in striking contrast to the science, discuss body weight as highly changeable. Yo-yo dieting is commonly described, as well as encroaching weight with pregnancy or after an injury. Marie sums up her experience this way:

> I have struggled with my weight all my life and I know I was a chubby kid. Certainly as a teenager I would say I was very overweight, got that under control and then I had a child and it's like now, it's just such an uphill battle.

Michelle articulates a similar experience:

> I had a weight issue when I was younger and then the way I managed that, I lost a lot of weight, by basically cutting out everything that

> I thought was a bad food and then depriving myself to the point where... there would be the binge cycle [...] It just started a cycle of, you know, losing and gaining.

In both cases the problem is not that the body cannot change – that a fat body stubbornly stays fat, that the brain of a fat subject is structured such that change is not possible. Instead, the body seems almost too changeable. Weight fluctuates up and down, and finding any stability comes, says Michelle, only with emotional changes and a less stringent outlook on eating and health:

> So that's why I am quite conscious of the fact of not having the right and wrong foods for my children. It's about having a balance, so I never had it as all or nothing, as either all the crap food or all the good food.

Because the interviews also covered childhood obesity, there was much discussion of children's bodies, and these accounts invariably treat the body as ontologically unstable rather than static. Children's bodies are of course always changing, as are their minds. Many participants resist the idea that a plump child must become an overweight or obese adult, and the measurement of children's bodies, particularly via the standard BMI measure, is frequently derided or condemned. Caroline, for example, describes an encounter with a maternal health nurse who

> measured and calculated and worked out [my daughter's BMI]. She said, 'Oh her BMI is a bit over, you need to...' and I just thought 'Oh', I thought '[how] bizarre, two years old and she is being measured for her BMI!'

In some cases this vigilance and the measurement it entails are framed as part of the problem, interrupting children's fragile developing healthy relationship to food. Marie acknowledges the need for healthy eating habits, but juxtaposes this need with the costs of emphasising the issue too much:

> [W]ith a small child I don't want to make too big a deal of it because you could send it the other way, you know [...and] then cause the very problem that you were trying to avoid. So it's very depressing [...] you think, no I don't want it to become everything because then it makes it a real psychological issue for someone, I think. If you're

> constantly on them about their weight then it does become their main focus in life because somebody has taught them that's all that matters.

It seems Marie seeks, as do many others, more balance than she believes the current climate of obesity enacts between monitoring health and living life free of potentially disruptive and counterproductive body image and eating concerns.

While it would not be accurate to say participants do not care about obesity at all, for themselves or for their children, or that they never treat the body as stable and intractable, the realities they constitute around body size, health and daily life cohere much more closely with the critical social science literature, with its doubts about the epidemiology, its awareness of the depth of meaning and significance of food and eating, and its interest in looking beyond 'fat' as self-evidently bad. As in the previous sections, a striking gap exists between the collateral realities made in the scientific discourse on overeating and obesity and those made in public discourse. Again, it seems unlikely that the realities made in the science – the coherence of addiction, the singularity of drugs, the simplicity of 'environment' and the stability of the body – will hold together well in public contexts any time soon.

Conclusion

In this chapter we traced the enactment of contemporary obesity realities in Australian women's accounts of food, eating and addiction. The aim in the first of the two chapters in this section of the book (Chapter 6) was to understand better how contemporary scientific accounts of obesity, those increasingly coming to shape public health responses and interventions, are remaking this phenomenon through the language of addiction, and in turn to consider how this movement of obesity into the domain of addiction is reshaping addiction itself. These aims were pursued through an analysis of four collateral realities made in the scientific literature on obesity – realities of addiction, drugs, the social and the body. Building on this, in the second chapter (Chapter 7) we explored public enactments of obesity and addiction, allowing comparison between the scientific and public realities currently under construction.

As we have demonstrated, the scientific account does not (yet) hold together beyond its own authorising context (and indeed, some debate and controversy remains there too, as will probably always be the case). Just as neuroaddiction models have yet to demonstrate any real benefits for the problem of drug addiction (Courtwright 2010), it is likely any such benefits will be equally slow, or slower, in coming for food addiction and obesity. Rather like the realities of drinking and alcohol addiction enacted in interviews with young people (discussed in Chapter 5), we find that the realities of eating, weight, the body and the social context of food enacted by the women in our study are, in many ways, more nuanced and convincing than those distilled in the science by the need to create overeating anew as a bounded, fixable problem. Indeed, they chime quite clearly with the sociological and feminist accounts outlined at the beginning of Chapter 6, in that they acknowledge that food, eating and weight are entirely embedded in (we might say made or enacted in) complex social circumstances and relations, including persistent binaries of gender, health and individual agency. While the difficulty with which the participants try to define addiction could be dismissed as an effect of the limits of their knowledge, again, as we argued in Chapter 5 in considering young people's articulations of alcohol addiction, this too would erase the very real confusion and controversy that characterises expert debate in the conventional addiction field. Instead, their struggles understandably enact the trickiness of addiction, the ambiguity of habit.

Will the gaps between scientific realities and public realities close any time soon? We have hinted at the answer to this question in acknowledging in this chapter and throughout the book the influence of scientific knowledges, their ability to marshal the epistemology and ontology of common sense realism to support their own institutional survival – to 'do' realities in particular ways and to wash away the messy processes by which this doing is done. It is possible that the language of neuroaddiction will move progressively into public discourse, even if the promises of the science were to remain unfulfilled. Yet this also depends upon practices of contestation. Whatever is not contested, whatever lies beyond the limits of contestability, Law says, works most powerfully to do the real. This analysis is one contribution to drawing back within the bounds of contestation four fundamentals of the new obesity and, in so doing, to contest the proliferating realities of neuroaddiction as well.

Conclusion

A Multiverse of Habits: 'Addicting' Science, Policy and Experience

In concluding this book, we wish to take quite seriously a question raised in Chapter 6 about the effects of scientising obesity as addiction. We asked about the fate of addiction in light of this relatively recent development, and the prospect that, surely, if overeating – something we are told many people do chronically – is a kind of addictive behaviour, addiction must be on the move from the margin to the centre. We are all, this development implies, not only potential addicts but already addicts in practice – classically intractable ones. We are chronically relapsing, dependent. It will probably come as no surprise by now that the authors of this book could not agree more. But of course, we embrace this idea for reasons rather far removed from those of the psychiatrists, neuroscientists, epidemiologists and even the majority of the sociologists, ethnographers and other cognate scholars who have addressed themselves to addiction. Those closest to us conceptually turn out, it seems, to be the many methamphetamine consumers, drinkers and mothers we spoke to in our research; not because they all shared a very specific critique of addiction, or even took up contemporary expert languages and labels alike. Their accounts varied in many ways; for example, we observed more alignment between experts and public in discussions of methamphetamine than of alcohol, and more in discussions of alcohol than of food. We can speculate as to why this might be, and one possible answer could be that the stronger the stigmatising of the substance, the less room individuals have to reject professional meaning-making about its consumption. Methamphetamine, as we have noted, is regularly demonised in the press, in policy and in service provision (where, for example, selective experiences among accident and emergency staff are given great prominence in public debate). Amid this variety in perspectives is, however, a noticeable thread – that of habit – and it is with habit that we wish to connect our final speculations on drugs and revisit our theoretical concerns. We think habit is more than just something humans *do* as they go about daily life. In line with the ideas about objects, subjects and assemblages we have taken up from the work of John Law and Bruno Latour, we think it *makes* humans and, further, *constitutes the nature of reality itself.*

In a lecture delivered to a group of graduate students in Russia in 2011, STS studies scholar Steve Woolgar outlined a series of provocative analytical moves of especial usefulness for projects such as ours. These moves allow seemingly irresistible, self-evident instances of scientific knowledge – hard facts, material objects (diseases, technologies, technical practices and so on) – to be subjected to critique to point to ways in which they 'could be otherwise' (Woolgar, 2011). Woolgar claims this motto, that things 'could be otherwise', as the key insight and driver of STS, forgetting, perhaps, its founding salience to many long-standing areas of research and thought, notably anthropological and feminist scholarship (including Carol Bacchi's critical analytical approach to reading policy and its problems on which we have drawn in this book). Still, it is a clarifying idea, prompting a range of questions about how best to analyse the 'mundane' (defined by Woolgar as both the unremarkable and, more pointedly, the taken for granted) to find out how they work, how they are constituted such that they are, indeed, taken for granted. Three of the analytic moves Woolgar recommends are, first, what he calls 'gerunding', after the grammatical practice that makes verbs act as nouns (adding 'ing' to self-evident concepts to foreground that they are *made*); the second is to speak of objects and their persons, rather than persons and their objects; and the third is, addressing John Law's (2004) notion of the 'hinterland' to concepts, practices and objects, to think not about how hinterlands shape objects but of how certain hinterlands come to be ascribed to objects in political processes.

The first of these analytic provocations describes rather neatly the project we have undertaken in this book. One of the examples Woolgar gives of 'gerunding' is that of the future. We shouldn't be analysing 'futures' he says. Instead, we should be analysing 'futuring', that is, how certain futures, and certain ideas and imperatives of the future, are made. This is an arresting example, filled with promise, but we appreciate our own even more. As we have argued throughout the book, addiction is not a thing that can be better or worse understood and measured and addressed. It is not an 'elephant', but not because it is a different animal. Rather it is an unstable assemblage made in practice and – an effect of politics – it is multiple and contingent, its shape, scale and content dependent upon a range of other equally labile phenomena. Setting aside that this is, of course, how all animals are anyway if we take our STS approach seriously, this assemblage is not so organised, coherent or coordinated to be mistaken for what we usually expect of a living animal. In so far as addiction, then, does not exist as a unified anterior object available to be studied, this book has been an act of 'addicting'. And we mean this, of course, in more ways than one. Most obviously, the book has explored the ways in which addiction is being made, that is, how the 'addicting' of contemporary neo-liberal societies and their subjects is going on. Substances, persons, brains and behaviours; the *DSM* and its lists; neuroscience and its scans and receptors, its endogenous opioids and cannabinoids; bread, chips and biscuits; drinking patterns, hangovers and regrets are all being made via addiction; they are all being brought into, or reinscribed in, particular overlapping but not identical ideas of addiction. Where Sedgwick (1993) saw an epidemic of 'addiction attribution', therefore, we see an epidemic of *addicting*, with all the material implications this revision suggests.

We understand this addicting, this making of addiction and the addicted, in a second sense too. Here another example Woolgar gives of gerunding acts as a useful pointer. Along with futuring, he invites us to think not of evidence but of 'evidencing'. This is an especially salient invitation for a domain of discourse so fraught and constrained in its processes of authorisation. The evidence, we see when we examine the addicting of methamphetamine via scientific and policy discourse in Chapter 2, is very obviously constituted from the weakest of orthodox resources. Unrefereed reports, journal articles and survey findings that do not quite support the claims the text accompanying the citation suggests they do, unreferenced assertions. Either we are so dependent upon the forcible constitution of methamphetamine as a demon drug that such questionable modes of 'evidencing' must emerge or – to take a broader view – we are so dependent upon the growing ideal of 'evidence-based policy' (Bell 2012) that despite the epistemological (not to mention ontological) limitations of evidence as it is currently constituted, we are obliged to present our mundane views of methamphetamine in the taken-for-granted modes of evidencing, that is, in the format of scientific knowledge. We are, in other words, addicted to more than drugs or food.

But here, in pointing out some particularly troubling addictions, we must take care. Our aim in this book has not been to lament the problem of addiction, hoping to help solve that 'terrible scourge' – to accept the moralities of addiction we find so much in need of critical scrutiny. We do not want to find better ways to eradicate heavy drinking (Australia's National Health and Medical Research Council 2009 guidelines warn against more than four standard drinks on any one occasion), or to help people say no to chocolate cake, to choose fruit instead on their birthdays, or better yet, vegetables since fruit too contains addicting sugars. We do not even aspire to offer alternatives to methamphetamine use, to insert 'meaning' into young people's lives such that they do not fall prey to 'drugs' and their instantly brain-altering, excessively rewarding effects. In short, we do not mean to present addiction as a problem in itself, even as we see some dependence, such as that on particular modes of evidencing, as problematic. Instead, we wish to make a double observation about the ubiquity of addiction, or as we propose, of *habit*.

What we have been doing in this book, and wish to make coalesce in this conclusion, is what Woolgar refers to as an 'ontography' and an 'epistemography' of addiction. We have not simply traced the rise of new knowledge about addiction, the discovery of new addictive substances and the biological processes by which addiction occurs. We have traced the way addiction is enacted into being, the kinds of being it is coming to be said to possess, and the modes and practices of knowledge making with which these ontologies are being established. Yes, when we speak of the ubiquity of addiction, we are referring to the sense in which assemblages of addiction are being mobilised to figure and act on an increasing number of activities and states. Daily life is being 'addicted', reframed via shifting notions of addiction, and in this book our aim has been to draw attention to this. More than this, however, our aim in this book has also been to draw attention to the wider implications of addiction, its place as repetition, and of repetition in change as well as stasis (Fraser & valentine 2008, as discussed in the Introduction), and to bring this set of associations into an encounter with some useful theoretical resources. As John Law (2011) says, drawing on Judith Butler's (1990, 1993) theory of gender performativity, reality is performative. And, as Judith Butler says, performativity is repetition. Gender exists, is stabilised and is understood to reflect an underlying reality of sex, only in the repetition of gendered acts. Likewise, we can say of realities more generally that they must be repeated if they are to hold stable, to become and stay real. We must do them over and over – we must addict ourselves to them if they are to appear to make a stable world filled with stable objects. This stable world and its stable objects are reciprocally dependent upon us to enact them through repetition. We could conclude, then, that all reality is addiction. But we would prefer to say all reality is habit. And here is the point at which we come back to the territory we share with the interview participants who offer such rich otherwises to the narrow addiction realities being enacted in our key addiction objects: methamphetamine, alcohol and food.

What do we mean by this notion of habit, and how does it differ from addiction? As each of the three sections on specific substances and their encounters with notions of addiction shows us, expert discourses are working, with varying degrees of success, to enact new addictions: addiction without withdrawal (methamphetamine), addiction without daily use (methamphetamine and alcohol) and addiction without an exceptionalist substance or recourse to a pathology of daily use (food). These addictions are enacted, however, as part of a project to constitute a singular addiction concept refined to fewer and fewer features and attributes (such as, for example, in the idea that the brain's reward system will eventually tell us all we need to know about curing addiction). In making addiction in these ways, expert discourses are also enacting a range of collateral realities: the stable anterior object that pre-exists our efforts to know it, agency as inhering in substances or vulnerable brains, drugs as a unified category, the social dimensions of drug use as narrowly conceived 'environment', the body as fixed and stable, and many more. These collateral realities are enacted in multiple overlapping ways across the three areas, and within the differing discursive contexts provided by the scientific literature, *DSM* debates and policy documents we explored.

The expert discourses of addiction also find their way in partial enactments, and to varying degrees, into our interviews with the people who in one way or another are the targets of such expertise. For this reason and for many others, we do not offer their words as an ideal alternative to the dissatisfactions thrown up by the expertise. At the same time, they tell us a great deal about the potential of habit as an otherwise to addiction. Whereas addiction is rigid, narrow and linear, habit is flexible, encompassing and diffuse. Addiction and habit both describe repetition and pattern, but only habit can recognise change, not as the end or antithesis of repetition but as part of it, entailed in it. This idea has long roots. Drawing on the work of influential French philosopher of habit Fèlix Ravaisson, whose key work on the subject, *On Habit*, was first published in 1838, David Bissell (2012, n.p.) describes habit as 'evidencing a dual logic of continuity and change'. Ravaisson, Bissell argues, uses habit to 'attend to the plasticity of bodies' (n.p.). This is just as we have conceived habit and the need to exceed the polarities presently animating addiction. In short, science and policy will never do justice to addiction assemblages and the way they change, emerge and subside, until they can see the multiplicity and instability that is as characteristic to them as is their continuity and stasis. Likewise, habit offers a way of understanding the ontological and epistemological commitments and practices of scientific enterprises and policymaking themselves, their repetitions (of orthodoxies of evidence, of narrow, linear causation, of the anteriority of reality) as well as their capacity for innovation and change.

Here Woolgar's comments about objects, persons and hinterlands are useful. Substances and subjects do not so much *have* hinterlands of knowledges, values and attributes (it is not easy, after all, to escape essentialism in such a formulation); instead they are *ascribed* hinterlands in acts of ontological politics. Addiction, science, policy and experience are all given different hinterlands at different times and these constrain our revisions and reimaginings. The commitments and practices of science and policy to which we just referred are part of such hinterlands. Somehow, and with time, however, these hinterlands change, and this book is one contribution to this process of change. Likewise, as Woolgar says, it is usual to speak of persons and their objects: the woman and her car and the way she drives it, you and your Facebook account and the events you describe and present on it, the young man and his slab of beer and how he drinks it. This is the habitual ascription of agency – from subject to object. But, as has so many times been emphasised in STS and its discussions of actor network theory, this habit does not do justice to the action of objects or the moralities of technologies (Latour 2002). Subjects, objects, actions. Repetition and rupture. Stabilisation and change. Addiction is, at present at least, too rigid and polarising for these inconvenient multiplicities, but habit is not.

In a 2004 article exploring new ways of thinking about the body after social constructionism and the rise of 'biopower' (the idea that subjects are being governed increasingly through their bodies), Latour makes a range of comments of use here. Criticising conventional science in favour of a version outlined by Isabelle Stengers, he discusses two things of value for our closing remarks on the uses of habit. Aiming to propose a way of talking about the body that exceeds essentialism *and* social constructionism, both of which he says ultimately leave science in charge of knowledge about the body, he argues that we should not think in terms of a universe made of essences, but of a 'multiverse made of habits' (2004, 213). By multiverse he means the universe 'freed from its premature unification' (213). This multiverse is part of a larger argument he makes, following Stengers, that a new standard for science must be developed which must, among other things, reject narrow notions of falsifiability, and pursue more courageous approaches to research that allow the enactment of knowledges and realities not already defined by the assumptions, techniques and questions built into the methods adopted. Good science, they both argue, is not reductive. It articulates differences instead of fixing facts. It builds more differences onto those already known instead of eliminating alternative versions and seeking to discount them via an authoritative claim to truth, 'bulldozing' its way through other disciplines, that is, declaring them obsolete. If scientists do science better in this way, Latour (2004, 213) argues, the result will not be multiple worlds with no hope of resolution, but *a multiverse,* a universe that has not been 'done on the cheap and without due process'.

Is addiction being done on the cheap and without due process? There is much in our interviews to suggest that something in this interpretation is worth attending to, even as we see certain debates continue within the sciences and between the sciences and other disciplines. Whether their subject be the much feared illicit substance (methamphetamine), the widely embraced if increasingly suspect symbol of the good life (alcohol) or the source of everyday nourishment (food), the interviews indicate a need to avoid premature unification. The bodies, practices, relationships and circumstances of consumption they articulate offer many, many differences left to comprehend and to add to what is taken already to be known. Here we might turn to Latour (2004, 222) again, where he describes this knowledge making, saying it forms part of the task of 'composing the common world'. This task cannot be done in haste. Instead, he says:

> [T]he proliferation of other enduring versions of what the multiverse is made of, even after some sciences have spoken, simply means... that the task of composing the common world has not been prematurely simplified. (2004, 222–3)

Whether or not composing such a common world is a task we, the authors of this book, agree should be pursued or has any hope of completion, we are taken by the recognition here of the importance of other enduring versions of reality and the need both Latour and Stengers identify to leave room for more than the versions traditional sciences are equipped and inclined to produce. Indeed, Latour, citing Stengers, specifies this need, saying the sciences must be more 'polite' when entering explanations into the 'composition of the common world'. As he puts it, 'No common world can be achieved if what is common has already been decided, by the scientists, out of sight of those whose "commonalities" are thus made up' (2004, 223).

It seems the sciences must adopt new habits, become more 'polite' about other ways of seeing and enacting the world (although 'politeness' seems a rather slight term for what is needed in enacting addiction differently and people diagnosed with it). Whatever its name, it seems we are all responsible for promoting this change given we are all responsible for accepting or rejecting the knowledges the sciences craft and promote. This can be done in many ways, but rejecting the universe of essences is perhaps the most pressing. When it comes to addiction, the implications of this are immediately apparent – indeed, the amusing example Latour gives at the close of his article of the scientist who carries a photograph of his wife's brain scan in his wallet, claiming it, we gather, as the essence of her, brings us neatly back to addiction neuroscience and the *DSM* and their knowledge-making habits. While both compete to define and respond to addiction, those whose commonalities are being made up are sidelined.

So long as the addicting of bodies, practices, substances and selves continues to expand, so too will the difficulty of constituting from all these phenomena, and holding stable, the universe of essences scientists (and policymakers, and service providers in turn) might hope to discover. As we have seen in this book, while addiction is expanding, it must pay a price to do so, and that is to relinquish some of its very essence (its hallmarks of withdrawal, tolerance, daily use and so on). This is necessary for addiction's 'institutional survival' (Law 2011). Other essences are, of course, identified in turn, and these (the difference between need and want, the place of occasional as well as regular consumption) are undergoing processes of stabilisation with varying degrees of success. As our focus throughout the book on collateral realities has sought to capture, some of this work is explicit – bulldozed in to remake addiction as the kind of problem it is thought possible to solve – but some is rarely noticed. It lies, as Law (2011) has said, beyond the bounds of contestability and has required examination to bring it back within these bounds. In the process of making food addictive, for example, obesity neuroscience is enacting very specific collateral realities of 'drugs' (as an essentialised category of substances all alike in effects), of drug addiction (as a homogenous state amenable to set treatment responses), of bodies (as fixed: fat or thin but rarely both over time) and of the lifeworlds of ordinary people (as 'obesogenic environments'). These collateral realities must be continually re-enacted. In this respect they are themselves habits, and will change just as surely as all repetition introduces change. In the meantime, these realities work to enact more and more individuals and their lives in particular modes of addiction, largely without their input.

This book could close on this note – a call to social scientists, policymakers, advocates and other interested parties to expect and create sciences, including social sciences, *of proliferating differences*, to resist the premature unification of the various kinds of consumption into a certain reality of addiction, to ask for and expect more epistemological politeness. There is much to be said for this call and the ontology of rich assemblages it recognises. As well as this, however, we wish to revisit once more the idea of habit as an otherwise to addiction, merely to repeat our suggestion that far from representing a state of being on the margins of normality, or an anomaly in the smooth, forward flow of life, or a stalling or detour in the proper progress and development of reality, habit is part and parcel of the normal, of life and of reality. If we do wish to take on the task of composing a common world, we might begin with habit: addiction as more subtly and generously and effectively understood as habit, addiction sciences, policy and public accounts and all their collateral realities as habit. And even reality itself as habit, made only in the repetition and dependence and contingency so familiar from the enactments of addiction we have made the subject of this book.

Appendix: Interview Data Collection Methods

Chapter 3

The consumer accounts of methamphetamine use analysed in Chapter 3 were collected in semi-structured, in-depth interviews and participant observation undertaken in Melbourne, Australia, in 2009 and 2010. They were collected during the ethnographic component of an ethno-epidemiological study investigating methamphetamine use and service provision. Thirty-one people (17 men, 13 women and one transgender woman; average and median age 36 years, range 22–56 years) were interviewed. All had taken methamphetamine at least once a week in the six months preceding the interview or on a regular basis prior to entering drug treatment. Twenty-six participants reported being born in Australia, with all but two identifying ethnically as Anglo or European. Four participants had attended a tertiary institution and three had completed secondary education. Four participants were employed full-time, with 20 in receipt of either a disability or unemployment pension, and 15 were enrolled in opioid substitution therapy. Interviews were conducted in cafes, parks, local services and private homes and lasted an average of one hour (range 27–128 minutes). Interviews were digitally recorded and professionally transcribed. Participants were reimbursed $30 for their time and out-of-pocket expenses in accordance with accepted practice in Australia (Fry & Dwyer 2001). Ethics approval for the research was granted by the Curtin University Human Research Ethics Committee (HR150/2007). The project was entitled 'Understanding the barriers to improved access, engagement and retention of methamphetamine users in health services' (National Health and Medical Research Council Project Grant 479208). We are extremely grateful to Robyn Dwyer for conducting the interviews and participant observation, and to the participants who so generously gave their time.

Chapter 5

The analysis conducted in Chapter 5 was based on semi-structured interviews conducted in 2012 in Melbourne, Australia, with 30 young adults aged between 18 and 24 years (15 men, 15 women). All participants had consumed at least one alcoholic drink within the previous six months. The majority of participants ($n = 23$) were either full- or part-time students. Nineteen were engaged in full- or part-time employment, and one participant was neither studying nor working. Fourteen were born outside Australia and 11 spoke another language in addition to English. Interviews were conducted in cafes, parks, educational settings and hotels. All research interviews were digitally recorded and professionally transcribed. Participants were reimbursed $40 for their time and out-of-pocket expenses in accordance with accepted practice in Australia. Ethics approval for the research was granted by the Curtin University Human Research

Ethics Committee (NDRI-02-2012). The project was entitled 'Understanding and reducing alcohol-related harm in urban settings: Opportunities for intervention' (Australian Research Council Linkage Project 100100017). We are extremely grateful to Mutsumi Karasaki and Christine Siokou for conducting the interviews, to Sarah MacLean for coding the interview transcripts and to the participants who so generously gave their time.

Chapter 7

The study on which our analysis in Chapter 7 was based involved 30 in-depth qualitative interviews conducted with mothers ($n = 24$) and childcare workers ($n = 6$) across three childcare sites in Victoria, Australia. The interviews were conducted in 2012. To recruit participants, flyers advertising the study were posted at each childcare site and circulated by managers of each of the childcare centres. Eight mothers and two childcare workers from each site were interviewed. The interviews were semi-structured in format, 60–90 minutes in length, and involved discussions about childhood obesity and experiences of managing and caring for the diet, health and weight of young children, and for the women themselves. The mothers all had pre-school-aged children and many also had older children aged up to 16 years. The interviews were transcribed verbatim, de-identified and analysed for major themes with the aid of NVivo data management software. The project team developed a coding framework when the dataset was complete based on key topics covered in the interviews and the strength of emerging themes. Sites in the inner Melbourne and greater Melbourne area were selected in order to recruit a socio-economically and culturally diverse range of participants for the study. Ethics approval for the research was granted by the Monash University Human Research Ethics Committee (CF11/693–2011000332). The project was entitled 'Improving Australia's response to childhood obesity: Prevention education and its impact on mothers and families' (Australian Research Council Discovery Project 110101759). We are extremely grateful to Claire Tanner, who conducted the interviews for this study, and to the participants who so generously gave their time.

Notes

1 Models of Addiction

1. DSM numbering underwent a change between the fourth and fifth editions, moving from Roman to Arabic (*DSM-IV* to *DSM-5*).
2. The WHO International Classification of Diseases (*ICD-10*) also contains a widely used diagnostic model of substance dependence which is similar to the *DSM* model (World Health Organization 1992). However, while the *ICD-10* is often used by governments in official coding, the *DSM* is more commonly used by mental health professionals and in research.
3. It should be noted that the *DSM-5* does state that 'prescription medications can be used inappropriately' and that a substance use disorder can be diagnosed in this situation if other symptoms of 'compulsive, drug-seeking behavior' are present, reflecting current concerns about prescription opiate abuse (APA 2013a, 484). However, the identification and interpretation of behaviour as compulsive and aberrant is itself enmeshed with judgements about character and moral worth, and influenced by the varying levels of surveillance faced by different types of patients (Bell & Salmon 2009; Keane 2013b).
4. According to the APA, the Roman numeral system was dropped for the *DSM-5* to make the manual 'more responsive to breakthroughs in research' by freeing diagnostic guidelines from a 'static publication date' (APA 2013c). Thus, incremental updates in the diagnostic criteria will be identified with a decimal, such as *DSM-5.1*, *DSM-5.2* and so on, until a whole new edition is required.

2 Stabilising Stimulants: Amphetamine Dependence and Methamphetamine Addiction

1. We return to these debates in Chapter 4.
2. This conceptualisation of addiction as a state – 'a real beast' – is similar to that offered by Leshner (2001): that is, that addiction is a 'different state of being' from non-addiction.
3. The *DSM-5* has opted for a dimensional framing: 'substance use disorders' (the re-introduced term for dependence) can be severe or moderate.
4. This definition of addiction (discussed in Chapter 1) appears in all of the NIDA publications cited earlier in the chapter.
5. Later in the 2002 report, tolerance is defined in more conventional terms.
6. The term 'tolerance' has been removed from this section in the 2006 report.
7. We can also see this march to bio-power in Schuckit's (2012, 521) lament that 'If... sensitive, specific, reliable, and valid biological criteria could be found,

there might be less room for disagreement regarding the best way to diagnose these [substance use] disorders'.

8. Interestingly, the authors cite NIDA as one of their funding sources.

3 Making Methamphetamine in Drug Policy and Consumer Accounts

1. The Australian policy documents almost exclusively use the term 'dependence' rather than 'addiction'.
2. Note: one of the authors of this book (Moore) was a member of the Research Reference Group that provided advice to the Project Management Group during the development of the national strategy. He provided confidential feedback on the draft strategy and background paper, which included some of the issues discussed in this chapter.
3. Note here the fudging of terminology about the relationship between drug use and harm: 'drug-related' is a vague description of this relationship whereas 'consequences' explicitly implies causation.
4. In this sense, the 2012 Strategy anticipates the terminology and ontology of the *DSM-5* (released in 2013), which also conceptualises addiction as a 'substance use disorder' that underlies behavioural problems.

4 A Field in Disarray? The Constitution of Alcohol Addiction in Expert Debates

1. See, for example, Room's (1984a) critique of 'problem deflation' in anthropological accounts of drinking.
2. This is a point we also made in Chapter 1 in relation to the 11 *DSM* criteria for the diagnosis of a 'substance use disorder'.
3. Ducci and Goldman (2008) provide a rare exception when they offer the following definition: 'Alcoholism is a chronic relapsing disorder'.
4. Note again the range and types of drinking included within a single claim.
5. Note how gender is invoked here as a risk factor whereas it is often ignored or downplayed.
6. The simplification of environment reaches its zenith when Ducci and Goldman claim (2008, 1420) that 'animal models are extremely useful because they offer the possibility of controlling environmental influences enhancing gene effects and eliminating confounds that might underlie correlations'.
7. Gender again seems to be important here.
8. See, for example, Li et al. (2007) and invited commentaries; and O'Brien (2011) and invited commentaries.
9. Perhaps unsurprisingly, given his earlier dismissal of Shaw's (1979) sociological critique of dependence, Edwards does not mention sociology in his list of useful disciplines.
10. For another example of addiction-as-elephant, see Kalant (1994).

6 Junk: The Neuroscience of Food Addiction and Obesity

1. Parts of this chapter were originally published as Fraser, S. (2013) Junk: Overeating and obesity and the neuroscience of addiction. *Addiction Research & Theory*, 21(6), 496–506.
2. This literature review and the section on fat and feminism that follows it are adapted from a more detailed discussion first published in Fraser, S., Maher, J., & Wright, J. (2010). Between bodies and collectivities: Articulating the action of emotion in obesity epidemic discourse. *Social Theory & Health,* 8(2), 192–209.

Bibliography

Adam, D. (2013). Mental health: On the spectrum. *Nature*, 496, 416–418.

Agrawal, A., & Lynskey, M. T. (2008). Are there genetic influences on addiction: Evidence from family, adoption and twin studies. *Addiction*, 103, 1069–1081.

American Psychiatric Association. (2000). *Diagnostic and statistical manual of mental disorders DSM-IV-TR*, Washington, DC: American Psychiatric Press.

American Psychiatric Association. (2013a). *Diagnostic and statistical manual of mental disorders DSM-5*, Washington, DC: American Psychiatric Press.

American Psychiatric Association. (2013b). *Substance-related and addictive disorders*, DSM-5 website. Retrieved from http://www.dsm5.org/Documents/Substance%20Use%20Disorder%20Fact%20Sheet.pdf.

American Psychiatric Association. (2013c). *Frequently asked questions, DSM-5 development*. Retrieved from http://www.dsm5.org/about/pages/faq.aspx.

American Society of Addiction Medicine. (2013). *Definition of addiction*. Retrieved from http://www.asam.org/for-the-public/definition-of-addiction.

Armstrong, E. (2007). Moral panic over meth. *Contemporary Justice Review*, 10(4), 427–442.

Australian National Council on Drugs. (2007). *Methamphetamines: Position paper*, Canberra: ANCD.

Ayres, T. C., & Jewkes, Y. (2012). The haunted spectacle of crystal meth: A media-created mythology? *Crime Media Culture, 8*(3), 315–332.

Babor, T. F., Caetano, R., Casswell, S., Edwards, G., Giesbrecht, N., Graham, K., Grube, J. W., Gruenewald, P., Hill, L., Holder, H., Homel, R., Österberg, E., Rehm, J., Room, R., & Rossow, I. (2001). *Alcohol: No ordinary commodity. Research and public policy*, Oxford: Oxford University Press.

Babor, T. F., Caetano, R., Casswell, S., Edwards, E., Giesbrecht, N., Graham, K., Grube, J. W., Hill, L., Holder, H., Homel, R., Livingston, M., Österberg, E., Rehm, J., Room, R., & Rossow, I. (2010). *Alcohol: No ordinary commodity: Research and public policy* (2nd ed.), Oxford: Oxford University Press.

Bacchi, C. (2009). *Analysing policy: What's the problem represented to be?* French's Forest: Pearson Education Australia.

Baker, A., Gowing, L., Lee, N. K., & Proudfoot, H. (2004). Psychosocial interventions for psychostimulant users. In A. Baker, N. K. Lee & L. Jenner (Eds.), *Models of intervention and care for psychostimulant users, 2nd Edition, National Drug Strategy monograph series no. 51* (pp. 63–84), Canberra: Australian Government Department of Health and Ageing.

Baker, A., Lee, N. K., Claire, M., Lewin, T. J., Grant, T., Pohlman, S., Saunders, J. B., Kay-Lambkin, F., Constable, P., Jenner, L., & Carr, V. J. (2005). Brief cognitive behavioural interventions for regular amphetamine users: A step in the right direction. *Addiction*, 100, 367–378.

Baker, A., Lee, N. K., & Jenner, L. (Eds.) (2004). *Models of intervention and care for psychostimulant users, 2nd Edition, National Drug Strategy monograph series No. 51,* Canberra: Australian Government Department of Health and Ageing.

Balding, J. (1997). *Young people and illegal drugs in 1996: A report based on data collected between 1987 and 1996 using the health related behaviour questionnaire.* Exeter: Exeter University Schools Health Education Unit.

Ball, D. (2008). Addiction science and its genetics. *Addiction*, 103, 360–367.

Balogh, S. (2009, April 19). Anti-drug ads rehashed for Rudd's $18 million campaign. *The Courier-Mail*. Retrieved from http://www.couriermail.com.au/news/features/more-anti-drug-ads/story-fn2mcu0g-1225702944780.

Barad, K. (2003). Posthumanist performativity: Toward an understanding of how matter comes to matter. *Signs: Journal of Women in Culture and Society*, 28(3), 801–831.

Bartu A., Freeman, N. C., Gawthorne, G. S., Codde, J. P., & Holman, C. D. (2004). Mortality in a cohort of opiate and amphetamine users in Perth, Western Australia. *Addiction*, 99, 53–60.

Becker, H. (1963). Becoming a marihuana user. In *Outsiders: Studies in the sociology of deviance*, New York, NY: The Free Press.

Bell, K. (2012). Cochrane reviews and the behavioural turn in evidence-based medicine. *Health Sociology Review*, 21(3), 313–321.

Bell, K., & Salmon, A. (2009). Pain, physical dependence and pseudoaddiction: Redefining addiction for 'nice' people? *International Journal of Drug Policy*, 20(2), 170–178.

Berridge, K. (2007). The debate over dopamine's role in reward. *Psychopharmacology*, 191(3), 391–431.

Berridge, V. (1999). *Opium and the people*, London: Free Association Books.

Bissell, D. (2012). Agitating the powers of habit: Towards a volatile politics of thought. *Theory and Event*, 15(1), 1–22.

Bordo, S. (1993). *Unbearable weight: Feminism, Western culture and the body*, Berkeley, Los Angeles and London: University of California Press.

Bourgois, P. (2000). Disciplining addictions: The bio-politics of methadone and heroin in the United States. *Culture, Medicine and Psychiatry*, 24(2), 165–95.

Bourgois, P., & Schonberg, J. (2009). *Righteous Dopefiend*, Berkeley, CA: University of California Press.

Boyd, S., & Carter, C. (2010). Methamphetamine discourse: Media, law, and policy. *Canadian Journal of Communication*, 35, 219–237.

Brown, R. A. (2010). Crystal methamphetamine use among American Indian and White youth in Appalachia: Social context, masculinity, and desistance. *Addiction Research and Theory*, 18(3), 250–269.

Brown, R., & Grey, M. (2012). The pedagogy of regret: Facebook, binge drinking and young women. *Continuum: Journal of Media and Cultural Studies*, 26(3), 357–369.

Buchman, D., Iles, J., & Reiner, P. (2010). The paradox of addiction neuroscience. *Neuroethics*, 4(2), 65–77.

Butler, J. (1990). *Gender trouble: Feminism and the subversion of identity*, New York and London: Routledge.

Butler, J. (1993). *Bodies that matter: On the discursive limits of sex*, New York and London: Routledge.

Caetano, R., & Babor, T. (2006). Diagnosis of alcohol dependence in epidemiological surveys: An epidemic of youthful alcohol dependence or a case of measurement error? *Addiction*, 101(s1), 111–114.

Campbell, N. (2007). *Discovering addiction: The science and politics of substance abuse research*, Ann Arbor, MI: University of Michigan Press.

Campbell, N. (2010). Toward a critical neuroscience of 'addiction'. *BioSocieties*, 5(1), 89–104.

Campbell, N. (2012). Medicalization or biomedicalization: Does the diseasing of addiction fit the frame? In J. Netherland (Ed.), *Critical perspectives on addiction* (pp. 3–25), New York, NY: Emerald.

Campos, P., Saguy, A., Ernsberger, P., Oliver, E., & Gaesser, G. (2005). The epidemiology of overweight and obesity: Public health crisis or moral panic? *International Journal of Epidemiology*, 35, 55–60.

Carnell, S., Cooke, L., Cheng, R., Robbins, A., & Wardle, J. (2011). Parental feeding behaviours and motivations. A qualitative study in mothers of UK pre-schoolers. *Appetite*, 57(3), 665–673.

Carr, E. S. (2010). *Scripting addiction: The politics of therapeutic talk and American sobriety*, Princeton, NJ: Princeton University Press.

Carter, A., & Hall, W. D. (2010). The need for more explanatory humility in addiction neurobiology. *Addiction*, 105(5), 790–791.

Charney, D. S., et al. (2002). Neuroscience agenda to guide development of a pathophysiologically based classification system. In D. Kupfer, M. First & D. Regier (Eds.), *A research agenda for DSM-V*, Washington, DC: American Psychiatric Association.

Churchill, A. C., Burgess, P. M., Pead, J., & Gill, T. (1993). Measurement of the severity of amphetamine dependence. *Addiction*, 88, 1335–1340.

Clatts, M. C., Welle, D. L., & Goldsamt, L. A. (2001). Reconceptualizing the interaction of drug and sexual risk among MSM speed users: Notes toward an ethno-epidemiology. *AIDS and Behavior*, 5(2), 115–130.

Cohen, S. (2002). *Folk devils and moral panics: The creation of the Mods and Rockers* (3rd ed.), London and New York: Routledge.

Compton, W., & Volkow, N. (2006). Abuse of prescription drugs and the risk of addiction. *Drug and Alcohol Dependence*, 83S, S4–S7.

Conrad, P., & Schneider, J. W. (1992). *Deviance and medicalization: From badness to sickness*, Philadelphia, PA: Temple University Press.

Cottler, L., Helzer, J. E., Mager, D., Spitznagel, E. L., & Compton, W. M. (1991). Agreement between DSM-III and III-R substance use disorders. *Drug and Alcohol Dependence*, 29(1), 17–25.

Courtwright, D. (2010). The NIDA brain disease paradigm: History, resistance and spinoffs. *BioSocieties*, 5(1), 137–147.

Davis, C. (2009). Psychobiological traits in the risk profile for overeating and weight gain. *International Journal of Obesity*, 33(S2), S49–53.

Davis, C., & Carter, J. (2009). Compulsive overeating as an addiction disorder: A review of theory and evidence. *Appetite*, 53, 1–8.

Davis, C., Zai, C., Levitan, R. D., Kaplan, A. S., Carter, J. S., Reid-Westoby, C., Curtis, C., Wight, K., & Kennedy, J. L. (2011). Opiates, overeating and obesity: A psychogenetic analysis. *International Journal of Obesity*, 35(10), 1347–1354.

Degenhardt, L., Roxburgh, A., & Black, E. (2003). *Cocaine and amphetamine mentions in accidental drug-induced deaths in Australia 1997–2003*, Sydney: National Drug and Alcohol Research Centre.

Deleuze, G., & Parnet, C. (2002). *Dialogues*. [1977]. Trans. Hugh Tomlinson and Barbara Habberjam. New York: Columbia University Press.

Denzin, K. (1987). *The alcoholic self*, London: Sage.
Department of Health and Ageing. (n.d.). *Introduction: National Amphetamine-Type Stimulant Strategy 2008–2011*. Retrieved from http://www.health.gov.au/internet/drugstrategy/publishing.nsf/Content/ats-strategy-08-l~ats-strategy-08-l-1~ats-strategy-08-l-1.3.
Department of Human Services. (2008). *Victorian Amphetamine-Type Stimulant (ATS) and Related Drugs Strategy 2009–2012*, Melbourne: Victorian Government Department of Human Services.
Derrida, J. (1993). The rhetoric of drugs. An interview. *Differences: A Journal of Feminist Cultural Studies*, 5(1), 1–25.
Deutscher, P. (2006). Repetition facility: Beauvoir on women's time. *Australian Feminist Studies*, 21(51), 327–342.
Division of Clinical Psychology (British Psychological Society). (2013). *DCP position statement on classification*. Retrieved from http://dcp.bps.org.uk/dcp/the_dcp/news/dcp-position-statement-on-classification.cfm.
Ducci, F., & Goldman, D. (2008). Genetic approaches to addiction: Genes and alcohol. *Addiction*, 103, 1414–1428.
Duff, C. (2005). Party drugs and party people: Examining the 'normalization' of recreational drug use in Melbourne, Australia. *International Journal of Drug Policy*, 16(3), 161–170.
Dumit, J. (2004). *Picturing personhood: Brain scans and biomedical identity*, Durham, NC: Duke University Press.
Edwards, G. (1980). Alcoholism treatment: Between guesswork and certainty. In G. Edwards & M. Grant (Eds.), *Alcoholism treatment in transition* (pp. 307–321), London: Croom Helm.
Edwards, G. (1986). The alcohol dependence syndrome: A concept as stimulus to enquiry. *British Journal of Addiction*, 81(2), 171–183.
Edwards, G. (2012). Letter to the editor: 'The evil genius of the habit': DSM-5 seen in historical context. *Journal of Studies on Alcohol and Drugs*, 73(4), 699–701.
Edwards, G., & Grant, M. (Eds.), (1980). *Alcoholism treatment in transition*, London: Croom Helm.
Edwards, G., & Gross, M. (1976). Alcohol dependence: Provisional description of a clinical syndrome. *British Medical Journal*, 1, 1058–1061.
Edwards, G., Arif, A., & Hodgson, R. (1984). Nomenclature and classification of drug- and alcohol-related problems: A shortened version of a WHO memorandum. *Australian Alcohol and Drug Review*, 3, 76–85.
Elam, M. (2012). Pharmaceutical incursion on cigarette smoking at the birth of the brain disease model of addiction. In J. Netherland (Ed.) *Critical perspectives on addiction* (pp. 53–75), Bingley: Emerald.
Ericksen, C., & Wilcox, R. (2006). Please, not 'addiction' in *DSM-V*. *American Journal of Psychiatry*, 163(11), 2015–2016.
Evans, B. (2006). Gluttony or sloth: Critical geographies of bodies and morality in (anti)obesity policy. *Area*, 38(3), 259–267.
First, M. (2010). Paradigm shifts and the development of the diagnostic and statistical manual of mental disorders. *La Revue Canadienne de Psychiatrie*, 55(11), 692–700.
Fraser, S. (2006). The chronotope of the queue: Methadone maintenance treatment and the production of time, space and subjects. *International Journal of Drug Policy*, 17(3), 192–202.

Fraser, S. (2010). Repetition and rupture: The gender of agency in methadone maintenance treatment. In C. Patton (Ed.), *Rebirth of the clinic: Places and agents in contemporary health care* (pp. 69–97), Minneapolis, MN: University of Minnesota Press.

Fraser, S. (2011). Beyond the 'potsherd': The role of injecting drug use-related stigma in shaping hepatitis C. In S. Fraser & D. Moore (Eds.), *The drug effect: Health, crime and society* (pp. 91–105), Melbourne: Cambridge University Press.

Fraser, S. (2013). Junk: Overeating and obesity and the neuroscience of addiction, *Addiction Research & Theory*, 21(6), 496–506.

Fraser, S., Maher, J., & Wright, J. (2010). Between bodies and collectivities: Articulating the action of emotion in obesity epidemic discourse. *Social Theory & Health*, 8(2), 192–209.

Fraser, S., & Moore, D. (2011). The drug effect: Constructing drugs and addiction. In S. Fraser & D. Moore (Eds.), *The drug effect: Health, crime and society* (pp. 1–16), Melbourne: Cambridge.

Fraser, S., & Seear, K. (2011). *Making disease, making citizens: The politics of hepatitis C*, Aldershot: Ashgate.

Fraser, S., & valentine, k. (2008). *Substance and substitution: Methadone subjects in liberal societies*, Basingstoke: Palgrave Macmillan.

Fry, M. L. (2010). Countering consumption in a culture of intoxication. *Journal of Marketing Management*, 26(13–14), 1279–1294.

Fry, C., & Dwyer, R. (2001). For love or money? An exploratory study of why injecting drug users participate in research. *Addiction*, 96(9), 1319–1325.

Gard, M., & Wright, J. (2001). Managing uncertainty: Obesity discourses and physical education in a risk society. *Studies in Philosophy & Education*, 20, 535–549.

Gearhardt, A. N., Grilo, C. M., DiLeone, R. J., Brownell, K. D., & Potenza, M. N. (2011). Can food be addictive? Public health and policy implications. *Addiction*, 106(7), 1208–1212.

Gomart, E. (2002). Methadone: Six effects in search of a substance. *Social Studies of Science*, 32(1), 93–135.

Gomart, E. (2004). Surprised by methadone: In praise of drug substitution treatment in a French clinic. *Body & Society*, 10(2–3), 85–110.

Goode, E., & Ben-Yehuda, N. (1994). Moral panics: Culture, politics, and social construction. *Annual Review of Sociology*, 20, 149–171.

Gossop, M., Griffiths, P., Powis, B., & Strang, J. (1992). Severity of dependence and route of administration of heroin, cocaine and amphetamines. *British Journal of Addiction*, 87, 1527–1536.

Halkitis, P. N., Fischgrund, B. N., & Parsons, J. T. (2005). Explanations for methamphetamine use among gay and bisexual men in New York City. *Substance Use and Misuse*, 40(9–10), 1331–1345.

Hart, C. L., Marvin, C. B., Silver, R., & Smith, E. E. (2012). Is cognitive functioning impaired in methamphetamine users? A critical review. *Neuropsychopharmacology*, 37(3), 586–608.

Hasin, D. (2012). Combining abuse and dependence in DSM-5. *Journal of Studies on Alcohol and Drugs*, 73(4), 702–704.

Hayes, L., Smart, D., Toumbourou, J.W., & Sanson, A. (2004). *Parenting influences on adolescent alcohol use*, Melbourne: Australian Institute of Family Studies.

Heimisdottir, J., Vilhjalmsson, R., Kristjansdottir, G., & Meyrowitsch, D. W. (2010). The social context of drunkenness in mid-adolescence. *Scandinavian Journal of Public Health*, 38(3), 291–298.

Hekman, S. (2010). *The material of knowledge: Feminist disclosures*, Bloomington, IN: Indiana University Press.

Hodgson, R., & Stockwell, T. (1985). The theoretical and empirical basis of the alcohol dependence model: A social learning perspective. In N. Heather, I. Robertson & P. Davies (Eds.), *The misuse of alcohol: Crucial issues in dependence treatment and prevention* (pp. 17–34), London: Croom Helm.

Hyman, S. (2005). Addiction: A disease of learning and memory. *The American Journal of Psychiatry*, 162(8), 1414–1422.

Hyman, S. (2007). Can neuroscience be integrated into the DSM-V? *Nature Reviews Neuroscience*, 8, 725–732.

Hyman, S. (2010). The diagnosis of mental disorders: The problem of reification. *Annual Review of Clinical Psychology*, 6, 155–179.

Hyman, S., & Malenka, C. (2001). Addiction and the brain: The neurobiology of compulsion and its persistence, *Nature Reviews Neuroscience*, 2, 695–703.

Ifland, J., Preuss, H., Marcus, M., Rourke, K., Taylor, W., Burau, K., et al. (2009). Refined food addiction: A classic substance use disorder. *Medical Hypotheses*, 72, 518–526.

Insel, T. (2013). Transforming diagnosis, *National Institute of Mental Health: Director's Blog*. Retrieved from http://www.nimh.nih.gov/about/director/2013/transforming-diagnosis

Järvinen, M., & Room, R. (2007). Youth drinking cultures: European experiences. In M. Järvinen & R. Room (Eds.), *Youth drinking cultures: European experiences* (pp. 1–17), Hampshire and Burlington: Ashgate.

Jayne, M., Valentine, G., & Holloway, S. L. (2010). Emotional, embodied and affective geographies of alcohol, drinking and drunkenness. *Transactions of the Institute of British Geographers*, 35(4): 540–554.

Jellinek, E. M. (1960). *The disease concept of alcoholism*, New Brunswick, NJ: Hillhouse Press.

Jenkins, P. (1994). 'The ice age': The social construction of a drug panic. *Justice Quarterly*, 11(1), 7–31.

Joe, K. A. (1996). Lives and times of Asian-Pacific American women drug users: An ethnographic study of their methamphetamine use. *Journal of Drug Issues*, 26(1), 199–218.

Jutel, A. (2011). Classification, disease and diagnosis. *Perspectives in Biology and Medicine*, 54(2): 189–205.

Kafka, M. (2010). Hypersexual disorder: A proposed diagnosis for DSM-V. *Archives of Sexual Behavior*, 39(2), 377–400.

Kalant, H. (1994). Comments on Edwards's editorial 'Addiction, reductionism and Aaron's rod'. *Addiction*, 89, 13–14.

Kalant, H. (2010). What neurobiology cannot tell us about addiction. *Addiction*, 105(5), 780–789.

Keane, H. (1999). Adventures of the addicted brain. *Australian Feminist Studies*, 14(29), 63–76.

Keane, H. (2000). Setting yourself free: Techniques of recovery. *Health*, 4(3), 324–345.

Keane, H. (2002). *What's wrong with addiction?* Melbourne: Melbourne University Press.

Keane, H. (2009). Foucault on methadone: Beyond biopower. *International Journal of Drug Policy*, 20(5), 450–452.

Keane, H. (2011). The politics of visibility: Drug users and the spaces of drug use. *International Journal of Drug Policy*, 22(6), 407–409.

Keane, H. (2013a) Making smokers different with nicotine: NRT and quitting. *International Journal of Drug Policy*, 24(3), 189–195.

Keane, H. (2013b). Categorising methadone: Addiction and analgesia. *International Journal of Drug Policy*. Retrieved from http://dx.doi.org/10.1016/j.drugpo.2013.05.007 (published online 13/6/13).

Keane, H., & Hamill, K. (2010). Variations in addiction: The molecular and the molar. *BioSocieties*, 5(1), 52–69.

Keane, H., Moore, D., & Fraser, S. (2011). Addiction and dependence: Making realities in the DSM. *Addiction*, 106(5), 875–877.

Kirk, S., & Kutchins, H. (1992). *The selling of DSM: The rhetoric of science in psychiatry*, New York, NY: Aldine de Gruyter.

Kirkland, A. (2011). The environmental account of obesity: A case for feminist skepticism. *Signs*, 36(2), 463–485.

Klee, H. (2001). Amphetamine use: Crystal gazing into the new millennium. Part one – What is driving demand? *Journal of Substance Use*, 6, 22–35.

Kloep, M., Hendry, L. B., Ingebrigtsen, J. E., Glendinning, A., & Espnes, G. A. (2001). Young people in 'drinking' societies? Norwegian, Scottish and Swedish adolescents' perceptions of alcohol use. *Health Education Research*, 16(3), 279–291.

Kozlowski, L., & Wilkinson, D. A. (1987). Use and misuse of the concept of craving by alcohol, tobacco and drug researchers. *British Journal of Addiction*, 82(1), 31–36.

Kunitz, S. J., & Levy, J. E. (1974). Changing ideas of alcohol use among Navaho Indians. *Quarterly Journal of Studies on Alcohol*, 35, 243–259.

Kupfer, D., First, M., & Regier, D. (Eds.) (2002). *A research agenda for DSM-V*, Washington, DC: American Psychiatric Association.

Kushner, H. (2006). Taking biology seriously: The next task for historians of addiction? *Bulletin of the History of Medicine*, 80(1), 114–143.

Kushner, H. (2010). Toward a cultural biology of addiction. *BioSocieties*, 5(1), 8–24.

Latour, B. (1993). *We have never been modern*, Cambridge: Harvard University Press.

Latour, B. (2002). Morality and technology: The end of the means (trans. Venn). *Theory, Culture & Society*, 19(5–6), 247–260.

Latour, B. (2004). How to talk about the body? The normative dimension of science studies. *Body & Society*, 10(2–3), 205–229.

Lauderback, D., & Waldorf, D. (1993). What ever happened to ice: The latest drug scare. *Journal of Drug Issues*, 23(4), 597–613.

Law, J. (2004). *After method: Mess in social science research*, London and New York: Routledge.

Law, J. (2011). Collateral Realities. In F. Dominguez Rubio & P. Baert (Eds.), *The politics of knowledge* (pp. 156–178), London: Routledge.

LeBesco, K., & Braziel, J. (2001). Introduction. In K. LeBesco & J. Braziel (Eds.), *Bodies out of bounds: Fatness and transgression* (pp. 1–15), Berkeley and London: University of California Press.

Lee, N. (2004). Risks associated with psychostimulant use. In A. Baker, N. Lee & L. Jenner (Eds.), *Models of intervention and care for psychostimulant users, 2nd Edition, National Drug Strategy monograph series no. 51* (pp. 51–59) Canberra: Australian Government Department of Health and Ageing.

Leland, J. (1976). *Firewater myths: North American Indian drinking and alcohol addiction*, New Brunswick, NJ: Rutgers Center of Alcohol Studies Monograph No. 11.

Lemert, E. (1951). *Social pathology*, New York, NY: McGraw-Hill.

Lende, D. H., Leonard, T., Sterk, C. E., & Elifson, K. (2007). Functional methamphetamine use: The insider's perspective. *Addiction Research and Theory*, 15(5), 465–477.

Leshner, A. (1997). Addiction is a brain disease, and it matters. *Science*, 278(5335), 45–46.

Leshner, A. (2001). Addiction is a brain disease. *Issues in Science and Technology*, XVII(3), 75–80.

Levine, H. G. (1978). The discovery of addiction: Changing conceptions of habitual drunkenness in America. *Journal of Studies on Alcohol and Drugs*, 39(1), 143–74.

Li, T.-K., Hewitt, B. G., & Grant, B. F. (2007). The alcohol dependence syndrome, 30 years later: A commentary. *Addiction*, 102, 1522–1530.

Lindsay, J. (2009). Young Australians and the staging of intoxication and self-control. *Journal of Youth Studies*, 12(4), 371–384.

Liu, Y., von Denee, K., Kobiessy, F., & Gold, M. (2010). Food addiction and obesity: Evidence from bench to bedside. *Journal of Psychoactive Drugs*, 42(2), 133–145.

Lobstein, T. (2006). Commentary: Obesity – public health crisis, moral panic or a human rights issue? *International Journal of Epidemiology*, 35, 74–76.

MacAndrew, C., & Edgerton, R. B. (1969). *Drunken comportment: A social explanation*, Chicago, IL: Aldine.

Manderson, D. (2011). Possessed: The unconscious law of drugs. In S. Fraser & D. Moore (Eds.), *The drug effect: Health, crime and society* (pp. 225–239), Cambridge: Cambridge University Press.

Marks, I. (1990). Behavioural (non-chemical) addictions. *British Journal of Addiction*, 85(11), 1389–1394.

Marshall, M. (1979). Introduction. In M. Marshall (Ed.), *Beliefs, behaviors, and alcoholic beverages: A cross-cultural survey* (pp. 1–11), Ann Arbor: University of Michigan Press.

Martin, C., Chung, T., & Langenbucher, J. (2008). How should we revise diagnostic criteria for substance use disorders in the DSM-V? *Journal of Abnormal Psychology*, 117(3), 561–575.

McCormick, M. (1969). First representations of the gamma alcoholic in the English novel. *Quarterly Journal of Studies on Alcohol*, 30, 957–980.

McKetin, R., McLaren, J., & Kelly, E. (2006). The relationship between crystalline methamphetamine use and dependence. *Drug and Alcohol Dependence*, 58, 198–204.

McKetin, R., McLaren, J., Kelly, E., Lubman, D., & Hides, L. (2006). The prevalence of psychotic symptoms among methamphetamine users. *Addiction*, 101, 1473–1478.

Measham, F. (2008). The turning tides of intoxication: Young people's drinking in Britain in the 2000's. *Health Education*, 108(3), 207–222.

Measham, F., & Brain, K. (2005). 'Binge' drinking, British alcohol policy and the new culture of intoxication. *Crime Media Culture*, 1(3), 262–283.

Merikangas, K. R., & Risch, N. (2003). Genomic priorities and public health. *Science*, 302, 599–601.

Mewton, L., Slade, T., McBride, O., Grove, R., & Teesson, M. (2011). An evaluation of the proposed DSM-5 alcohol use disorder criteria using Australian national data. *Addiction*, 106(5), 941–950.

Miller, P., O'Reilly, J. & Jarvis, M. (2010). News and notes: Study shows compulsive eating shares addictive biochemical mechanism with cocaine and heroin abuse. *Addiction*, 105, 1131–1134.

Ministerial Council on Drug Strategy. (2008). *National Amphetamine-Type Stimulant Strategy 2008–2011*, Canberra: MCDS.

Mol, A. (1999). Ontological politics: A word and some questions. In J. Law & J. Hassard (Eds.), *Actor network theory and after* (pp. 74–89), Oxford: Blackwell and the Sociological Review.

Monaghan, L. (2005). Discussion piece: A critical take on the obesity debate. *Social Theory and Health*, 3, 302–314.

Moore, D. (1992). Deconstructing 'dependence': An ethnographic critique of an influential concept. *Contemporary Drug Problems*, 19(3), 459–490.

Moore, D. (2009). 'Workers', 'clients' and the struggle over needs: Understanding encounters between service providers and street-based injecting drug users in an Australian city. *Social Science and Medicine*, 68(6), 1161–1168.

Moore, D. (2011). The ontological politics of knowledge production: Qualitative research in the multidisciplinary drug field. In S. Fraser & D. Moore (Eds.) *The drug effect: Health, crime and society* (pp. 73–88.). Melbourne: Cambridge University Press.

Moore, D., & Fraser, S. (2006). Putting at risk what we know: Reflecting on the drug-using subject in harm reduction and its political implications. *Social Science and Medicine*, 62(12), 3035–3047.

Murray, S. (2005). Doing politics or selling out? Living the fat body. *Women's Studies*, 34(3–4), 265–277.

Myslobodsky, M. (2003). Gourmand savants and environmental determinants of obesity. *Obesity Reviews*, 4, 121–128.

National Health and Medical Research Council. (2009). *Australian guidelines to reduce health risks from drinking alcohol*, Canberra: Commonwealth Printing Service.

National Institute on Drug Abuse. (2002). *Methamphetamine Abuse and Addiction* (Research Report Series), NIH Publication Number 02–4210, Rockville, NIDA.

National Institute on Drug Abuse. (2006a). *Methamphetamine abuse and addiction* (Research report Series), NIH Publication Number 02–4210, Rockville, MD: NIDA.

National Institute on Drug Abuse. (2006b). *Mind over matter: The brain's response to methamphetamine*, NIH Publication Number 06–4394, Rockville, MD: NIDA.

National Institute on Drug Abuse. (2007). *Drugs, brains, and behavior: The science of addiction*. Bethesda, MD: National Institutes of Health.

National Institute on Drug Abuse. (2010a). *Methamphetamine* (NIDA InfoFacts), Rockville, MD: NIDA.

National Institute on Drug Abuse. (2010b). *Drugs, brains, and behavior: The science of addiction*, Rockville, MD: NIDA.

Netherland, J. (2012). *Critical perspectives on addiction*, Bingley: Emerald.

Ning, A. M. (2005). Games of truth: rethinking conformity and resistance in narratives of heroin recovery. *Medical Anthropology*, 24, 349–382.

Nutt, D. (2009). Equasy: An overlooked addiction with implications for the current debate on drug harms. *Journal of Psychopharmacology*, 23(1), 3–5.

O' Brien, C. (2011). Addiction and dependence in DSM-V. *Addiction*, 106(5), 866–867.

O'Brien, C. (2012). Rationale for changes in DSM-5. *Journal of Studies on Alcohol and Drugs*, 73(4), 705.

O'Brien, C., Volkow, N., & Li, T. (2006a). What's in a word?: Addiction versus dependence in DSM-V. *American Journal of Psychiatry*, 163(5), 764–765.

O'Brien, C. Volkow, N., & Li, T. (2006b). Dr O'Brien replies. *American Journal of Psychiatry*, 163(11), 2016–2017.

Office of National Drug Control Policy. (2012). *National Drug Control Strategy 2012*, Washington, DC: Executive Office of the President of the United States.

Orford, J. (1985). *Excessive appetites: A psychological view of addictions*, Chichester: Wiley.

Orford, J. (2001). Addiction as excessive appetite. *Addiction*, 96(1), 15–31.

Parr, J., & Rasmussen, N. (2012). Making addicts of the fat. In J. Netherland (Ed.), *Critical perspectives on addiction* (pp. 181–200), Bingley: Emerald.

Pedersen, W., & Skrondal, A. (1998). Alcohol consumption debut: Predictors and consequences. *Journal of Studies on Alcohol and Drugs*, 59(1), 32–42.

Pelchat, M. (2009). Food addiction in humans. *The Journal of Nutrition*, 139(3), 620–622.

Potenza, M. (2008). The neurobiology of pathological gambling and drug addiction. *Philosophical Transactions of the Royal Society B*, 363(1507), 3181–3189.

Probyn. E. (2008). Silences behind the mantra: Critiquing feminist fat. *Feminism and Psychology*, 18(3), 401–404.

Quintero, G. (2012). Problematizing 'drugs': A cultural assessment of recreational pharmaceutical use among young adults in the United States. *Contemporary Drug Problems*, 39(3), 491–536.

Race, K. (2009). *Pleasure Consuming Medicine*, Durham, NC: Duke University Press.

Radio Iowa. (2005, 25 March). *Governor says 'meth epidemic' worse than terrorist threat.* Retrieved from http://www.radioiowa.com/2005/03/25/governor-says-meth-epidemic-worse-than-terrorist-threat/.

Ravaisson, F. (2009 [1838]). *Of habit.* Trans. C. Carlisle & M. Sinclair, London: Continuum.

Reinarman, C. (2005). Addiction as accomplishment: The discursive construction of disease. *Addiction Research & Theory*, 13(4), 307–320.

Reith, G. (2004). Consumption and its discontents. *British Journal of Sociology*, 55(2), 283–300.

Rhodes, T., Lilly, R., Fernandez, C., Giorgino, E., Kemmesis, U. E., Ossebaard, H. C., Lalam, N., Faasen, I., & Spannow, K. E. (2003). Risk factors associated with drug use: The importance of risk environment. *Drugs: Education, Prevention & Policy*, 10(4), 303–329.

Rich, E., & Evans, J. (2005). 'Fat ethics': The obesity discourse and body politics. *Social Theory and Health*, 3, 341–358.
Ritter, A., & Lintzeris, N. (2004). Specialist interventions in treating clients with alcohol and drug problems. In M. Hamilton, T. King, & A. Ritter (Eds.), *Drug use in Australia: Preventing harm* (pp. 221–235), South Melbourne: Oxford University Press.
Robinson, T. E., & Berridge, K. C. (2003). Addiction. *Annual Reviews in Psychology*, 54, 25–53.
Rogers, P., & Smit, H. (2000). Food craving and food 'addiction': A critical review of the evidence from a biopsychosocial perspective. *Pharmacology Biochemistry and Behavior*, 66(1), 3–14.
Room, R. (1983). Sociological aspects of the disease concept of alcoholism. In R. G. Smart (Ed.), *Research advances in alcohol and drug problems* (pp. 47–91), London and New York: Plenum Press.
Room, R. (1984a). Alcohol and ethnography: A case of problem deflation? *Current Anthropology*, 25(2), 169–191.
Room, R. (1984b). Alcohol problems and the sociological constructivist approach: Quagmire or path forward? Revised from a paper presented at the Alcohol Epidemiology Section Meetings of the International Council on Alcohol and Addictions, 4–8 June 1984, Edinburgh, Scotland. Retrieved from www.robinroom.net/quagmire.pdf.
Room, R. (1985). Dependence and society. *British Journal of Addiction*, 80(2), 133–139.
Room, R. (1987). *Social dimensions of alcohol dependence*, Berkeley, CA: Alcohol Research Group, Medical Research Institute of San Francisco.
Room, R. (1998). Alcohol and drug disorders in the international classification of disease: A shifting kaleidoscope. *Drug and Alcohol Review*, 17(3), 305–317.
Room, R. (2001). Governing images in public discourse about problematic drinking. In N. Heather, T. Peters & T. Stockwell (Eds.), *Handbook of alcohol dependence and alcohol-related problems* (pp. 33–45), Chichester: John Wiley & Sons.
Room, R. (2003). The cultural framing of addiction. *Janus Head*, 6(2), 221–234.
Room, R., Janca, A., Bennett, L., Schmidt, L., & Sartorius, N. (1996). WHO cross-cultural applicability research on diagnosis and assessment of substance use disorders. *Addiction*, 91(2), 199–220.
Rose, N. (1989). *Governing the soul: The shaping of the private self*, London: Routledge.
Rose, N. (2003). The neurochemical self and its anomalies. In R. Ericson & A. Doyle (Eds.), *Risk and morality* (pp. 407–437), Toronto: University of Toronto Press.
Rose, N. (2007). *The politics of life itself: Biomedicine, power, and subjectivity in the twenty-first century*. Princeton, NJ: Princeton University Press.
Russell, M. A. H. (1976). What is dependence? In G. Edwards, M. A. H. Russell, D. Hawks & M. MacCafferty (Eds.), *Drugs and drug dependence* (pp. 182–187), Lexington, KY: Lexington Books.
Safe, M., & Sager, M. (1990, May 26–27). Ice: The new vice. *Weekend Australian*, 8–14.
Saguy, A., & Riley, K. (2005) Weighing both sides: Morality, mortality, and framing contests over obesity. *Journal of Health Politics, Policy & Law*, 30(5), 869–923.

Schuckit, M. (2012). Editorial in reply to the comments of Griffith Edwards. *Journal of Studies on Alcohol and Drugs*, 73(4), 521–522.

Seddon, T. (2010). *A history of drugs: Drugs and freedom in the liberal age*, London: Routledge.

Sedgwick, E. (1993). Epidemics of the will. In E. Sedgwick, *Tendencies* (pp. 130–142), Durham, NC: Duke University Press.

Shaffer, H., LaPlante, D. A., LaBrie, R. A., Kidman, R. C., Donato, A. N., & Stanton, M. V. (2004). Toward a syndrome model of addiction. *Harvard Review of Psychiatry*, 12(6), 367–374.

Sharkey, P. (2007). Survival and death in New Orleans: An empirical look at the human impact of Katrina. *Journal of Black Studies*, 37(4), 482–501.

Shaw, S. (1979). A critique of the concept of the alcohol dependence syndrome. *British Journal of Addiction*, 74, 339–348.

Shaw, S. (1985). The disease concept of dependence. In N. Heather, I. Robertson & P. Davies (Eds.), *The misuse of alcohol: Crucial issues in dependence treatment and prevention* (pp. 35–44), London: Croom Helm.

Skinner, M., & Aubin, H. (2010). Craving's place in addiction theory. *Neuroscience and Biobehavioral Reviews*, 34, 606–623.

Slavin, S. (2004). Crystal methamphetamine use among gay men in Sydney. *Contemporary Drug Problems*, 31(3), 425–465.

Smith, C. (2011). A users' guide to juice bars and liquid handcuffs. *Space and Culture*, 15(1), 291–309.

Socialstyrelsen. (1997). Levnadsvanor och livsvillkor Socialstyrelsen [Living habits and living conditions]. *Folkhälsorapport*, Report Stockholm.

Solomon, R. (1977). An opponent process theory of acquired motivation. In J. Maser & M. Seligman (Eds.), *Psychopathology: Experimental models* (pp. 66–103), San Francisco: Freeman.

Stephenson, R. H., & Banet-Weiser, S. (2007). Super-sized kids: Obesity, children, moral panic, and the media. In J. Bryant (Ed.), *The children's television community* (pp. 277–291), Mahwah, New Jersey and London: Lawrance Erlbaum Associates.

Sussman, S., Lisha, N., & Griffiths, M. (2011). Prevalence of the addictions. *Evaluation & the Health Professions*, 34(4), 3–56.

Thomas, S. L., Hyde, J., Karunaratne, A., Herbert, D., & Komesaroff, P. A. (2008). Being 'fat' in today's world: A qualitative study of the lived experiences of people with obesity in Australia. *Health Expectations*, 11, 321–330.

Thorley, A. (1985). The limitations of the alcohol dependence syndrome in multidisciplinary service development. In N. Heather, I. Robertson & P. Davies (Eds.), *The misuse of alcohol: Crucial issues in dependence treatment & prevention* (pp. 72–94), London: Croom Helm.

Topp, L. (2006). Focusing on methamphetamines. *Of Substance*, 4(3), 10–13.

Topp, L., Kaye, S., Bruno, R., Longo, M., Williams, P., O'Reilly, B., Fry, C., Rose, G., & Darke, S. (2002). *Australian drug trends 2001: Findings of the Illicit Drug Reporting System (IDRS). NDARC monograph number 48,* Sydney: National Drug and Alcohol Research Centre.

Topp, L., Lovibond, P. F., & Mattick, R. P. (1998). Cue reactivity in dependent amphetamine users: Can monistic conditioning theories improve our understanding of reactivity? *Drug and Alcohol Review*, 17, 277–288.

Topp, L., & Mattick, R. P. (1997a). Validation of the amphetamine dependence syndrome and the SAmDQ. *Addiction*, 92(2), 151–162.

Topp, L., & Mattick, R. P. (1997b). Choosing a cut-off on the Severity of Dependence Scale (SDS) for amphetamine users. *Addiction*, 92(7), 839–845.

Topp, L., Mattick, R. P., & Lovibond, P. F. (1995). The nature of the amphetamine dependence syndrome: Appetitive or aversive motivation? *NDARC Technical Report No. 30*, Sydney: National Drug and Alcohol Research Centre.

Totaro, P. (2005, December 1). Ice party drug creates a new wave of addiction. *Sydney Morning Herald.* Retrieved from www.smh.com.au/news/national/ice-party-drug-creates-a-new-wave-of-addiction/2005/11/30/1133311107155.html.

Underwood, E. (2013). NIMH won't follow psychiatry 'bible' anymore. *Science Insider.* Retrieved from http://news.sciencemag.org/2013/05/nimh-wont-follow-psychiatry-bible-anymore.

Urbina, I. (2012, May 11). Addiction diagnoses may rise under guideline changes. *The New York Times.* Retrieved from www.nytimes.com/2012/05/12/us/dsm-revisions-may-sharply-increase-addiction-diagnoses.html?pagewanted=all&_r=0.

Valverde, M. (1998). *Diseases of the will: Alcohol and the dilemmas of freedom*, Cambridge: Cambridge University Press.

Valverde, M., & White-Mair, K. (1999). 'One day at a time' and other slogans for everyday life. *Sociology*, 33(2), 393–410.

Van der Zwaluw, C. S., & Engels, R. C. M. E. (2009). Gene-environment interactions and alcohol use and dependence: Current status and future challenges. *Addiction*, 104, 907–914.

Vitellone, N. (2010). Just another night in the shooting gallery? The syringe, space and affect. *Environment and Planning D*, 28(5), 867–880.

Volkow, N., & Li, T. (2004). Drug addiction: The neurobiology of behaviour gone awry. *Nature Reviews Neuroscience*, 5, 963–970.

Volkow, N., & O' Brien, C. (2007). Issues for DSM-V: Should obesity be included as a brain disorder? *The American Journal of Psychiatry*, 164(5), 708–710.

Volkow, N., & Wise, R. (2005). How can drug addiction help us understand obesity? *Nature Neuroscience*, 8(5), 555–560.

Vrecko, S. (2010a). 'Civilizing technologies' and the control of deviance. *Biosocieties*, 5(1), 36–51.

Vrecko, S. (2010b). Birth of a brain disease: Science, the state and addiction neuropolitics. *History of Human Sciences*, 23(52), 52–67.

Wakefield, J. (2006). Clarifying the distinction between disorder and nondisorder. In K. Phillips, M. First & H. Pincus (Eds.), *Advancing DSM: Dilemmas in psychiatric diagnosis* (pp. 23–56), Washington, DC: American Psychiatric Association.

Waldorf, D., Reinarman, C., & Murphy, S. (1991). *Cocaine changes: The experience of using and quitting*, Philadelphia, PA: Temple University Press.

Warhol, R., & Michie, H. (1996) Twelve step teleology: Narratives of recovery/recovery of narrative. In S. Smith & J. Watson (Eds.), *Getting a life: Everyday uses of autobiography* (pp. 327–350), Minneapolis: University of Minnesota Press.

Weaver, M. (2010). Medical sequelae of addiction. In D. Brizer & R. Castaneda (Eds.), *Clinical addiction psychiatry* (pp. 23–36), Cambridge: Cambridge University Press.

Weinberg, D. (2002). On the embodiment of addiction. *Body & Society*, 8(4), 1–19.

Weinberg, D. (2011). Sociological perspectives on addiction, *Sociology Compass*, 5(4), 298–310.

WHO Expert Committee on Drug Dependence. (1993). *WHO expert committee on drug dependence: 28th Report*, WHO Technical Report Series 836, Geneva: World Health Organization.

Wodak, A. (2007). Ethics and drug policy. *Psychiatry*, 6(2), 59–62.

Wood, E. (2010). Editorial: Evidence based policy for illicit drugs. *BMJ*, 341, c3374.

Woolgar, S. (2011). Where Did All the Provocation Go? – reflections on the fate of Laboratory Life. *STS Workshop at the European University of St Petersburg, Russia, 19th November 2011*. Retrieved from http://anthem-group.net/2013/08/09/reflections-on-the-fate-of-laboratory-life-woolgar/

World Health Organization. (1992). *The ICD-10 classification of diseases and related health problems*, Geneva: World Health Organization.

World Health Organization. (2004). *Neuroscience of psychoactive substance use and dependence*, Geneva: World Health Organization.

Yancey, A., Leslie, J., & Abel, E. (2006). Obesity at the crossroads: Feminist and public health perspectives. *Signs*, 31(2), 425–443.

Zinberg, N. E. (1984). *Drug, set, and setting*, New Haven, CT: Yale University Press.

Zule, W. A., & Desmond, D. P. (1999). An ethnographic comparison of HIV risk behaviors among heroin and methamphetamine injectors. *The American Journal of Drug and Alcohol Abuse*, 25(1), 1–23.

Index

Note: The letter 'n' following locators refers to notes

Manufactured by Amazon.ca
Acheson, AB